Complete I-CBT Manual

Inference-Based Cognitive Behavioral Therapy for OCD

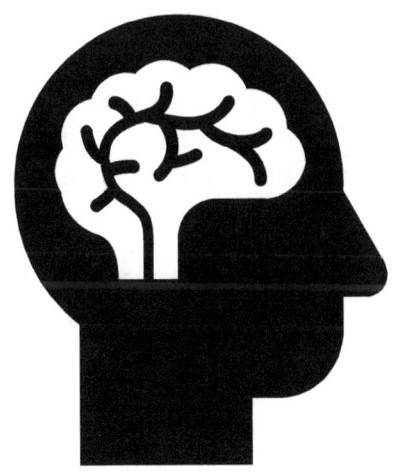

Theo Leonard Green.

© 2024 Theo Leonard Green. All rights reserved.

First Edition

ISBN: 978-1-923604-66-7

This book is intended for educational and informational purposes only and is designed for qualified mental health professionals. The content is not intended to be a substitute for professional medical advice, diagnosis, or treatment. Always seek the advice of qualified mental health professionals regarding any questions you may have about mental health conditions or treatment approaches.

The case studies presented in this book are fictional composites created for educational purposes. Any resemblance to actual persons, living or deceased, is purely coincidental. Names including but not limited to Sarah, Marcus, Elena, Jennifer, David, Robert, Lisa, Michael, Maria, James, Maya, Rebecca, Dr Chen, Dr. Martinez Thomas, Carlos, Grace, Amin, Miguel, and all other client names including therapist mentioned are fictional and used solely for illustrative purposes.

The author and publisher make no representations or warranties about the accuracy, completeness, or suitability of the information contained in this book. The information is provided "as is" without warranty of any kind. The author and publisher shall not be liable for any damages arising from the use of this information.

References to organizations, training programs, websites, and professional resources are provided for informational purposes only and do not constitute endorsement by the author or publisher.

Inference-Based Cognitive Behavioral Therapy (I-CBT) should only be practiced by appropriately trained and licensed mental health professionals. Proper training, supervision, and ongoing competency development are essential for safe and effective implementation.

About the Author

Theo Leonard Green is a registered mental health practitioner with over a decade of experience in forensic settings, criminal justice services, and various mental health institutions. His clinical background spans correctional facilities, psychiatric units, and community mental health centers, providing him with extensive experience treating across diverse populations.

Table of Contents

About the Author 1
Chapter 1: I-CBT and the Reasoning Revolution in OCD Treatment 4
Chapter 2: Historical Development and Key Figures 15
Chapter 3: Theoretical Foundations and the Inference-Based Model 27
Chapter 4: I-CBT and Traditional CBT Approaches 42
Chapter 5: OCD Through the I-CBT Lens 64
Chapter 6: The Inference Chain Model and Obsessional Sequences 80
Chapter 7: Obsessional Doubt - The Cornerstone of I-CBT 92
Chapter 8: Primary and Secondary Inferences in Clinical Practice 103
Chapter 9: Reasoning Biases and the Tricks of OCD 114
Chapter 10: Reality Sensing and Sensory Information 125
Chapter 11: Clinical Assessment in I-CBT 138
Chapter 12: Case Conceptualization Using the I-CBT Framework 153
Chapter 13: Differential Diagnosis and Treatment Selection 169
Chapter 14: Treatment Structure and the 12-Module Protocol 185
Chapter 15: Modules 1-3 - Understanding the Obsessional Sequence 198
Chapter 16: Modules 4-6 - Vulnerable Self and Imagination 211
Chapter 17: Modules 7-9 - Reality Sensing and Alternative Narratives .. 226
Chapter 18: Modules 10-12 - Consolidation and Relapse Prevention 238
Chapter 19: Advanced Techniques and Special Considerations 252
Chapter 20: Training Requirements and Competency Development 265
Chapter 21: Ethical and Professional Considerations 284
Appendix A: Clinical Forms and Assessments 318
Appendix B: Client Handouts and Psychoeducation Materials 325

Appendix C: Case Studies and Clinical Examples 343
Appendix D: Training Resources and References 358
Reference 367

Chapter 1: I-CBT and the Reasoning Revolution in OCD Treatment

Sarah sits across from me, her hands clasped tightly in her lap. She's already been through two rounds of traditional therapy for her contamination fears, complete with exposure exercises and anxiety management techniques. Yet here she is again, struggling with the same thoughts that won't leave her alone.

"I know it doesn't make sense," she tells me, frustration evident in her voice. "I know the doorknob isn't really contaminated. I know washing my hands twenty times won't actually protect my family. But knowing doesn't seem to matter. The thoughts keep coming anyway."

Sarah's story captures something important that traditional approaches to OCD often miss. She has all the rational knowledge she needs. She can explain why her fears are unrealistic. She's practiced exposure exercises and learned coping strategies. But none of this addresses the real problem: her mind keeps creating doubt where none should exist.

This is where Inference-based Cognitive Behavioral Therapy changes everything.

Sarah's Contamination Obsessions Despite "Knowing Better"

Sarah is thirty-two, works as an accountant, and considers herself a logical person. She came to therapy because her contamination fears were taking over her life, despite her clear understanding that they made no rational sense.

Her day begins at 5:30 AM with a forty-five-minute shower routine. She washes each part of her body in a specific order, repeating if she "doesn't feel clean enough." After showering, she needs another twenty minutes to get dressed because touching her clean body with potentially contaminated clothing creates new doubts.

The kitchen presents daily challenges. Sarah can't use the coffee maker without extensive cleaning because "what if someone touched it with dirty hands?" She knows her husband is clean, knows he washed his hands, but the possibility that he might have missed something creates an avalanche of doubt.

At work, Sarah avoids the bathroom until absolutely necessary. Public restrooms feel like minefields of contamination. She's developed elaborate strategies for opening doors, flushing toilets, and washing hands that leave her exhausted before her workday even begins.

"The worst part," Sarah explains, "is that I can see how crazy this looks. I'm not stupid. I understand germs and hygiene. I know most bacteria won't hurt me. But my brain just won't accept that information."

Traditional CBT helped Sarah understand her anxiety patterns and taught her relaxation techniques. Exposure therapy gradually introduced her to feared situations. She learned to tolerate touching doorknobs and shaking hands. But the fundamental problem remained: her mind continued generating doubt about contamination, and she couldn't figure out why.

This is exactly the kind of case where I-CBT offers something different. Rather than focusing on Sarah's anxiety or trying to reduce her fears through exposure, I-CBT looks at how her mind creates doubt in the first place. It asks a different question: Why does Sarah's brain keep telling her she might be contaminated when all the evidence says otherwise?

The Paradigm Shift from Anxiety Disorder to Reasoning Disorder

For decades, mental health professionals have understood OCD as an anxiety disorder. This makes intuitive sense - people with OCD feel anxious, their symptoms seem driven by fear, and they engage in compulsions to reduce anxiety. The anxiety model has guided treatment approaches that focus on reducing fear responses and helping people tolerate anxiety without engaging in compulsions.

But research by O'Connor and Aardema published in the Journal of Anxiety Disorders suggests that this anxiety-focused view misses the real mechanism driving OCD. Their comprehensive review of the inference-based approach demonstrates that OCD might be better understood as a reasoning disorder - a problem with how people process information and draw conclusions, rather than simply a problem with anxiety.

This shift changes everything about how we understand and treat OCD.

The Traditional Anxiety Model suggests that people with OCD:

- Experience intrusive thoughts that create anxiety
- Perform compulsions to reduce anxiety
- Avoid situations that trigger anxiety
- Need exposure therapy to learn that anxiety decreases naturally
- Benefit from anxiety management techniques

The I-CBT Reasoning Model proposes that people with OCD:

- Generate doubts through faulty reasoning processes
- Perform compulsions to resolve doubt (not anxiety)
- Avoid situations that trigger reasoning confusion
- Need to learn better reasoning skills
- Benefit from addressing the doubt-creation process directly

This isn't just a subtle difference in terminology. It represents a fundamental shift in how we understand what's actually happening in the minds of people with OCD.

Sarah's case illustrates this perfectly. Her problem isn't that she's too anxious about germs - she's generating doubt about contamination through faulty reasoning processes. Her mind takes perfectly normal situations (touching a doorknob) and creates elaborate stories about possible contamination that have no basis in reality.

Research published in the Journal of Affective Disorders by Aardema and O'Connor found that people with OCD don't actually have higher baseline anxiety than other people. What they have is a tendency to create doubt through specific reasoning errors. They take remote possibilities and treat them as probable realities. They focus on what might be true rather than what the evidence actually shows.

Why Traditional Approaches Sometimes Fall Short

Traditional CBT for OCD has helped many people, and I don't want to minimize its benefits. Exposure and Response Prevention (ERP) therapy has strong research support and has provided relief for countless individuals struggling with obsessions and compulsions.

But here's the thing: traditional approaches sometimes miss the mark because they're addressing the wrong target.

When you focus only on anxiety, you miss the reasoning problems that create the anxiety in the first place.

Sarah's experience with traditional therapy shows this clearly. She learned to tolerate anxiety in contamination situations. She practiced touching doorknobs and not washing her hands immediately. She could sit with the discomfort and wait for her anxiety to decrease.

But she never learned why her mind kept creating contamination doubts. She never understood the reasoning processes that made her believe she might be contaminated when all evidence suggested otherwise. So while she could manage her anxiety better, the doubt-generating machine in her head kept running.

This creates several problems:

High Dropout Rates: Many people find exposure therapy too difficult and discontinue treatment. A study published in Clinical Psychology Review found that dropout rates for ERP can be as high as thirty percent, often because people find the anxiety-provoking exercises overwhelming.

Partial Response: Even successful ERP treatment often leaves residual symptoms. People learn to function better but continue experiencing intrusive thoughts and doubts.

Relapse Risk: Without addressing the underlying reasoning problems, people remain vulnerable to symptom return during stressful periods.

Treatment Resistance: Some individuals don't respond well to exposure-based approaches, leaving them with limited treatment options.

Sarah fell into the "partial response" category. Traditional therapy helped her function better at work and home, but she continued experiencing contamination thoughts daily. She could resist some compulsions but still spent significant mental energy battling doubts that felt compelling despite her rational knowledge.

"I kept thinking I was doing something wrong," Sarah recalls. "My therapist said the anxiety would decrease if I just kept practicing exposure. But the thoughts themselves never went away. I started to wonder if this was just how my brain worked."

I-CBT's Unique Contribution to the Field

I-CBT offers something genuinely different: it addresses the reasoning processes that create obsessional doubt in the first place.

Instead of asking "How can we reduce your anxiety about contamination?" I-CBT asks "Why does your mind keep creating doubt about contamination when there's no evidence to support it?"

This approach, developed through decades of research at the Institut universitaire en santé mentale de Montréal, focuses on what researchers call **inferential confusion** - the tendency to treat imagined possibilities as if they were realistic probabilities.

Research published in Psychotherapy and Psychosomatics by O'Connor and colleagues demonstrates that I-CBT can be as effective as traditional CBT for treating OCD, with some important advantages:

Higher Acceptability: People often find I-CBT more tolerable because it doesn't require deliberate exposure to anxiety-provoking situations.

Better Understanding: Clients report that I-CBT helps them understand why their minds create obsessional thoughts, rather than just how to cope with them.

Reduced Shame: By framing OCD as a reasoning problem rather than an anxiety problem, I-CBT can reduce the self-criticism many people feel about their symptoms.

Broader Application: I-CBT techniques can help with various forms of obsessional thinking, not just specific phobias addressed through exposure.

The approach works by helping people:

1. **Recognize** when they're engaging in obsessional reasoning
2. **Understand** how these reasoning processes create doubt
3. **Develop** skills for staying connected to sensory reality
4. **Create** alternative stories based on actual evidence

5. **Build** confidence in their ability to distinguish real from imagined threats

Sarah's treatment with I-CBT looked completely different from her previous therapy experiences. Instead of practicing touching contaminated objects, we explored how her mind created contamination stories. We examined the reasoning processes that took her from "I touched a doorknob" to "I might be contaminated and could harm my family."

"It was like learning about a magic trick," Sarah explains. "Once I understood how my mind was creating these doubts, they stopped seeming so convincing. I could see the reasoning errors happening in real time."

This isn't about dismissing anxiety or pretending that exposure therapy doesn't work. Both approaches have value, and some people benefit from combining elements of each. But I-CBT offers a fundamentally different way of understanding and addressing obsessional thinking that can be especially helpful for people who haven't responded well to traditional approaches.

How This Manual Is Structured for Optimal Learning

This manual takes you through I-CBT in a specific sequence designed to build your understanding progressively. You can't really master the treatment techniques until you understand the underlying theory, and you can't apply the theory effectively until you see how it works in practice.

We'll start with the foundations - the history, theory, and basic concepts that make I-CBT different from other approaches. Then we'll move into practical application, showing you how to assess clients, plan treatment, and implement specific interventions.

Here's what you can expect:

Part I: Foundations and Theory establishes the groundwork. You'll learn about I-CBT's development, its theoretical foundations, and how it differs from traditional CBT approaches. These chapters might feel abstract at first, but they're essential for understanding why I-CBT techniques work.

Part II: Core Principles and Clinical Concepts gets more specific about how obsessional thinking actually works. You'll learn about inference chains, reasoning biases, and the role of doubt in maintaining OCD symptoms.

Part III: Assessment and Case Formulation teaches you how to evaluate clients for I-CBT treatment and develop effective treatment plans based on their specific reasoning patterns.

Part IV: Treatment Protocol and Techniques provides detailed guidance for implementing I-CBT interventions. These are the practical skills you'll use in session with clients.

Part V: Professional Development and Implementation addresses the business side of I-CBT practice, including training requirements, ethical considerations, and building an I-CBT practice.

Each chapter includes:

- Learning objectives that tell you exactly what you should understand by the end
- Detailed case examples that show concepts in action
- Practice exercises that help you apply what you're learning
- Self-assessment questions to check your understanding
- References to current research supporting each concept

You'll notice that case examples appear throughout multiple chapters. Sarah, whom you met at the beginning of this chapter, will reappear as we explore different aspects of I-CBT theory and treatment. This repetition is intentional - it helps you see how different concepts connect and how they apply to real clinical situations.

Self-Assessment: Understanding Your Current Knowledge Base

Before we go further, it's helpful to assess your current understanding of OCD and its treatment. This isn't a test - it's a way to identify areas where you might need to pay special attention as we move through the material.

Take a moment to consider these questions:

About OCD in General:

- How would you currently explain what causes OCD symptoms?
- What role do you think anxiety plays in maintaining obsessional thinking?
- How do you understand the relationship between obsessions and compulsions?

About Treatment Approaches:

- What treatments for OCD are you familiar with?
- How do you think exposure therapy works to reduce OCD symptoms?
- What challenges have you observed with traditional OCD treatments?

About Reasoning and Thinking:

- How do you distinguish between realistic and unrealistic thoughts?
- What role do you think reasoning processes play in emotional problems?
- How might faulty reasoning contribute to psychological symptoms?

About Your Own Thinking:

- Can you think of times when you've worried about something despite having no real evidence for concern?
- How do you typically resolve doubts or uncertainties in your daily life?
- What helps you distinguish between possible and probable outcomes?

Your answers to these questions will influence how you absorb the material in this manual. If you're already familiar with CBT principles, some concepts will feel familiar while others might challenge your existing understanding. If you're new to therapy approaches altogether, everything might feel novel.

Neither background is better or worse for learning I-CBT. Experienced therapists bring valuable clinical skills but might need to adjust their thinking about how OCD works. New therapists have fewer preconceptions to overcome but need to develop foundational therapy skills alongside I-CBT-specific techniques.

The key is approaching this material with what researchers call a "beginner's mind" - openness to new ways of understanding familiar problems. Even if you've treated hundreds of people with OCD using traditional methods, I-CBT offers perspectives that might surprise you.

What You've Learned and What's Coming Next

OCD treatment is evolving. While anxiety-based approaches have helped many people, they don't address the reasoning processes that create obsessional doubt in the first place. I-CBT offers a different way of understanding and treating OCD that focuses on how people generate doubt rather than how they manage anxiety.

Sarah's story illustrates both the limitations of traditional approaches and the potential of I-CBT. Her "knowing better" didn't help because her problem wasn't a lack of knowledge - it was a reasoning process that kept creating doubt despite evidence to the contrary.

You're about to learn a treatment approach that:

- Views OCD as a reasoning disorder rather than an anxiety disorder
- Addresses the doubt-creation process directly
- Helps people understand why their minds generate obsessional thoughts
- Can be more tolerable than exposure-based approaches
- Offers hope for people who haven't responded well to traditional treatments

In the next chapter, we'll explore how I-CBT developed from clinical observations in Montreal to become a recognized treatment approach with growing research support. You'll meet the key figures who developed these ideas and learn how their insights changed our understanding of obsessional thinking.

But first, take a moment to consider how this new perspective on OCD might change your approach to treatment. What would it mean for your clients if their problem isn't anxiety that needs to be managed, but reasoning processes that can be corrected?

That shift in thinking - from anxiety management to reasoning correction - is at the heart of everything we'll explore in this manual. It's a simple change in perspective that can transform how you understand and treat one of the most challenging psychological conditions.

The reasoning revolution in OCD treatment starts with recognizing that people like Sarah aren't failing at anxiety management. They're succeeding at faulty reasoning. Once we understand that distinction, everything else becomes possible.

Chapter 2: Historical Development and Key Figures

The year was 1995, and Kieron O'Connor was growing frustrated. As a researcher at the Institut universitaire en santé mentale de Montréal, he'd been treating people with OCD using the best available methods - exposure therapy, anxiety management, cognitive restructuring. Many clients improved, but something bothered him about the approach.

"Why do we keep focusing on anxiety," he wondered, "when these people keep talking about doubt?"

This question would spark a research program that fundamentally changed how we understand obsessional thinking.

O'Connor noticed that his most challenging clients weren't necessarily the most anxious ones. They were the ones who couldn't stop creating doubt about situations that clearly posed no real threat. They would touch a clean doorknob and somehow convince themselves they might be contaminated. They would lock their front door and immediately doubt whether they'd actually turned the key.

These weren't anxiety problems in the traditional sense. They were reasoning problems.

The Montreal Origins: Kieron O'Connor and the IUSMM Team

Kieron O'Connor arrived in Montreal in the early 1990s with a background in experimental psychology and a growing interest in how people with OCD think differently from others. Unlike many researchers who focused on brain chemistry or behavioral patterns, O'Connor was fascinated by the mental processes that created obsessional thoughts in the first place.

The Institut universitaire en santé mentale de Montréal provided the perfect environment for this research. As one of Canada's leading psychiatric research centers, the IUSMM encouraged innovative approaches to understanding mental health conditions. O'Connor assembled a team of researchers who shared his curiosity about the cognitive mechanisms underlying OCD.

The team included Frederick Aardema, who would become O'Connor's key collaborator and eventual successor in developing I-CBT theory. Aardema brought expertise in phenomenological psychology - the study of conscious experience and how people make sense of their world. This philosophical background would prove crucial for understanding how people with OCD create doubt where none should exist.

Marie-Claude Pélissier joined the research team as they began developing assessment tools and treatment protocols. Her clinical expertise helped translate theoretical insights into practical interventions that could be used in therapy sessions.

But the real catalyst for I-CBT's development came from listening to clients describe their experiences in their own words.

"Traditional therapy kept telling me to challenge my anxious thoughts," one client explained to O'Connor. "But I wasn't anxious about contamination - I was convinced I was contaminated. The problem wasn't fear, it was that my mind kept creating these elaborate stories about how I might have been exposed to germs."

This distinction between fear and conviction became central to I-CBT theory. People with OCD weren't just afraid of contamination - they were generating beliefs about contamination through faulty reasoning processes.

O'Connor's team began studying exactly how these beliefs formed. They observed that people with OCD would start with minimal sensory information (touching a doorknob) and then construct elaborate narratives about what this might mean (the doorknob could have been touched by someone with dirty hands, who might have had a cold, which could spread to my family, causing serious illness).

The reasoning process moved from "I touched something" to "I might be contaminated" without any evidence supporting the connection. This wasn't anxiety - this was what the team began calling **inferential confusion**.

Evolution from Clinical Observation to Theoretical Framework

The development of I-CBT theory followed a pattern common in scientific discovery: careful observation leading to hypothesis formation, followed by systematic testing and refinement.

Phase 1: Clinical Observation (1995-1999) O'Connor and his team began documenting the specific reasoning patterns they observed in clients with OCD. They noticed that people with contamination obsessions didn't actually avoid germs more than other people - they avoided *doubt* about contamination. People with checking compulsions weren't more forgetful than others - they doubted their memory of completing tasks.

This led to a crucial insight: OCD symptoms seemed designed to resolve doubt rather than reduce anxiety.

Phase 2: Theoretical Development (2000-2005) The team began developing a formal theory about how obsessional thinking works. They proposed that people with OCD engage in what they called "inverse inference" - starting with a feared outcome and reasoning backward to find ways it might be possible.

Normal reasoning follows this pattern:

- Observation: "I see evidence of a threat"
- Conclusion: "Therefore, I might be in danger"

Obsessional reasoning reverses this:

- Fear: "I might be in danger"

- Reasoning: "What evidence could support this possibility?"

This backward reasoning process allows people to find "evidence" for almost any feared outcome, no matter how unlikely.

Phase 3: Treatment Development (2005-2010) With a theoretical framework in place, the team began developing specific interventions to address inferential confusion. Rather than challenging the content of obsessional thoughts, they focused on the reasoning processes that created these thoughts.

They developed techniques to help people:

- Recognize when they were engaging in obsessional reasoning
- Distinguish between sensory reality and imagination
- Create alternative stories based on actual evidence
- Build confidence in their ability to assess real vs. imagined threats

Phase 4: Empirical Testing (2010-2015) O'Connor's team conducted several controlled studies comparing I-CBT to traditional CBT approaches. Their research, published in journals like Cognitive Behaviour Therapy and the Journal of Anxiety Disorders, demonstrated that I-CBT could be as effective as exposure therapy while being more acceptable to many clients.

Phase 5: Refinement and Dissemination (2015-2019) As evidence for I-CBT's effectiveness grew, the team refined their treatment protocols and began training other therapists in the approach. They developed standardized assessment tools, treatment manuals, and training programs.

Seminal Publications: From the 1995 Paper to Contemporary Works

The evolution of I-CBT theory can be traced through key publications that built upon each other over more than two decades.

"Inference processes in obsessive-compulsive disorder: Some clinical observations" (1995) This paper, published in Behaviour Research and Therapy, represented O'Connor's first attempt to articulate why traditional approaches to OCD might be missing something important. He argued that people with OCD weren't simply responding to intrusive thoughts - they were actively creating doubt through specific reasoning processes.

The paper didn't propose a complete alternative to existing treatments, but it raised questions that would drive decades of subsequent research.

"A cognitive approach to obsessive compulsive disorder" (2003) Published in Cognitive and Behavioral Practice, this paper began outlining the specific reasoning errors that characterize obsessional thinking. O'Connor and Aardema identified several key patterns:

- **Categorical errors**: Treating possibilities as probabilities
- **Irrelevant associations**: Connecting unrelated events
- **Inverse inference**: Reasoning backward from feared outcomes
- **Out-of-context reasoning**: Applying information inappropriately

"Beyond Reasonable Doubt: Reasoning Processes in Obsessive-Compulsive Disorder and Related Disorders" (2008) This book, co-authored by O'Connor, Aardema, and Pélissier, presented the first comprehensive theory of I-CBT. It included detailed case studies, assessment tools, and treatment protocols that therapists could use in practice.

The book established I-CBT as a legitimate alternative to traditional CBT approaches and provided the foundation for subsequent research and development.

"The inference-based approach to obsessive-compulsive disorder: A comprehensive review" (2016) Published in the Journal of Affective Disorders, this review paper by Aardema and O'Connor synthesized more than two decades of research on I-CBT. It demonstrated that the approach had solid empirical support and could be considered an evidence-based treatment for OCD.

"Inference-Based Cognitive Behavioral Therapy versus Cognitive Behavioral Therapy for Obsessive-Compulsive Disorder: A Multisite Randomized Controlled Non-Inferiority Trial" (2024) This recent study, published in Psychotherapy and Psychosomatics, provided the strongest evidence yet for I-CBT's effectiveness. The randomized controlled trial found that I-CBT was as effective as traditional CBT for treating OCD, with some advantages in terms of treatment acceptability and client satisfaction.

The Phenomenological Roots: Edmund Husserl's Influence

To understand I-CBT fully, you need to appreciate its philosophical foundations in phenomenology - the study of conscious experience and how people make sense of their world.

Edmund Husserl, the founder of phenomenological philosophy, was interested in how people construct their understanding of reality through direct experience. He argued that we don't simply observe the world objectively - we actively interpret our experiences and create meaning from them.

This insight became crucial for understanding obsessional thinking.

Husserl distinguished between different types of mental acts:

- **Perception**: Direct sensory experience of the world
- **Imagination**: Mental representation of things not directly experienced
- **Memory**: Recollection of past experiences
- **Inference**: Drawing conclusions based on available information

In normal thinking, people maintain clear distinctions between these different mental processes. They know the difference between what they're actually seeing and what they're imagining might be there.

People with OCD, according to I-CBT theory, lose this distinction. They treat imagined possibilities as if they were perceived realities. They confuse what might be true with what they have evidence for.

Aardema's background in phenomenological psychology helped the Montreal team understand this confusion more precisely. He recognized that people with OCD weren't simply having intrusive thoughts - they were engaging in what Husserl would call "category errors," confusing different types of mental experience.

This philosophical framework provided important insights for treatment development. If the problem was confusion between imagination and perception, then treatment should focus on helping people distinguish between these different types of experience.

Frederick Aardema's Continuing Development Post-2019

Kieron O'Connor passed away in 2019, but his work continues through Frederick Aardema and other researchers who have carried forward I-CBT development.

Aardema has expanded I-CBT theory in several important directions:

Digital Age Applications: Aardema has explored how I-CBT principles apply to modern concerns like social media anxiety and information overload. He's shown that the same reasoning processes that create traditional OCD symptoms can also generate doubt about online interactions and digital information.

Cultural Adaptations: Research has begun examining how I-CBT can be adapted for different cultural contexts. The basic principles of distinguishing imagination from reality appear universal, but the specific content of obsessional thoughts varies across cultures.

Comorbidity Applications: Aardema and colleagues have investigated how I-CBT techniques can help with conditions beyond

OCD, including body dysmorphic disorder, health anxiety, and certain types of depression that involve obsessional thinking.

Neuroscience Integration: Recent research has begun examining the brain mechanisms underlying inferential confusion, providing biological support for I-CBT's psychological theories.

Training and Dissemination: Aardema has developed comprehensive training programs for therapists learning I-CBT, including online resources and certification programs that make the approach more widely available.

The work continues to evolve, with new research expanding our understanding of how reasoning processes contribute to psychological symptoms and how I-CBT techniques can address these problems.

Interactive Timeline of I-CBT Milestones

Understanding I-CBT's development helps you appreciate both its solid research foundation and its continued evolution. Here are the key milestones:

1995: O'Connor publishes first paper questioning anxiety-focused approaches to OCD

1998: Research team at IUSMM begins systematic study of reasoning processes in OCD

2001: First controlled study comparing I-CBT to traditional CBT approaches

2003: Development of Inferential Confusion Questionnaire (ICQ) assessment tool

2005: Publication of first treatment manual for I-CBT interventions

2008: "Beyond Reasonable Doubt" book establishes comprehensive I-CBT theory

2010: International OCD Foundation recognizes I-CBT as evidence-based treatment

2012: First training workshops offered outside Montreal

2015: Online training platform launches, making I-CBT education more accessible

2016: Comprehensive review confirms I-CBT's empirical support

2019: O'Connor's death marks transition to next generation of researchers

2021: COVID-19 pandemic leads to increased interest in I-CBT's telehealth applications

2024: Largest randomized controlled trial to date confirms I-CBT's effectiveness

This timeline shows that I-CBT isn't a new or untested approach - it represents more than twenty-five years of careful research and development by some of the world's leading OCD researchers.

Practice Exercise: Identifying Historical Influences in Current Practice

To help you understand how I-CBT's historical development influences current practice, try this exercise:

Think about a client you've worked with (or a case example you're familiar with) who has OCD symptoms. Consider how different historical perspectives might understand their presentation:

1990s Anxiety Model: How would traditional CBT from the 1990s conceptualize this case? What interventions would it suggest?

Early 2000s Cognitive Model: How did the cognitive revolution in CBT change understanding of this case? What new interventions became available?

2010s I-CBT Model: How does the inference-based approach change your understanding of what's happening for this client?

Current Integrated Approach: How might you combine insights from different historical periods to create the most effective treatment plan?

This exercise helps you see that I-CBT didn't develop in isolation - it built upon and refined earlier approaches while offering genuinely new insights about the nature of obsessional thinking.

What This History Means for Your Practice

The historical development of I-CBT teaches several important lessons for therapists learning this approach:

Scientific Foundation: I-CBT isn't based on a single study or theoretical speculation - it represents decades of careful research by multiple investigators. This gives you confidence that the approach has solid scientific support.

Clinical Origins: The theory developed from careful observation of real clients in real therapy sessions. This means I-CBT techniques are designed to address problems that actually occur in clinical practice, not just theoretical constructs.

Evolutionary Process: I-CBT theory has been refined and improved over time based on new research and clinical experience. This means you're learning an approach that continues to evolve and improve.

International Recognition: Major professional organizations now recognize I-CBT as an evidence-based treatment for OCD. This gives you confidence in recommending the approach to clients and colleagues.

Continuing Development: Research on I-CBT continues, with new applications and refinements being developed. This means your skills in this approach will remain current and valuable throughout your career.

Understanding this history also helps you explain I-CBT to clients and colleagues. You can describe it as an established, well-researched approach that offers a unique perspective on obsessional thinking, rather than an experimental or unproven technique.

Theory into Practice

The history of I-CBT shows how careful observation and systematic research can lead to breakthrough insights about psychological problems. O'Connor's simple question - "Why do we focus on anxiety when clients talk about doubt?" - sparked decades of research that changed how we understand and treat OCD.

In the next chapter, we'll explore the theoretical foundations that emerged from this historical development. You'll learn exactly what inferential confusion means, how it differs from normal reasoning, and why addressing reasoning processes can be more effective than managing anxiety for many people with OCD.

The story of I-CBT's development reminds us that good therapy is built on good observation. The researchers who developed this approach succeeded because they listened carefully to what their clients were actually experiencing, rather than assuming that existing theories explained everything.

As you learn I-CBT techniques, keep this spirit of careful observation alive in your own practice. Notice what your clients tell you about their reasoning processes. Pay attention to how they create doubt and what helps them distinguish between realistic and unrealistic concerns.

The history of I-CBT suggests that the next breakthrough in understanding obsessional thinking might come from a therapist like you, working with clients and noticing something that doesn't quite fit with existing theories.

Chapter 3: Theoretical Foundations and the Inference-Based Model

Maria sits in her car outside the grocery store, engine running, hands gripping the steering wheel. She's been here for fifteen minutes, unable to make herself go inside. Not because she's afraid of crowds or social interaction, but because her mind is spinning an increasingly elaborate story about what might happen.

"What if I accidentally knock something over and it breaks? What if the clerk thinks I'm stealing? What if I touch something contaminated and bring germs home to my children?"

None of these concerns are based on anything Maria has observed. She hasn't seen broken items, suspicious clerks, or obvious contamination. Her mind is simply generating these possibilities and then treating them as if they were real threats requiring immediate attention.

This is *inferential confusion* in action - the core mechanism that I-CBT identifies as the heart of obsessional thinking.

Understanding Inferential Confusion as the Core Mechanism

Inferential confusion refers to the tendency to treat imagined possibilities as if they were realistic probabilities. It's the mental process that takes a person from "I'm going to the store" to "I might cause a disaster" without any evidence supporting the connection.

To understand inferential confusion, you need to understand how normal inference works first.

Normal Inference Process:

1. **Observation**: "I see evidence in the environment"

2. **Reasoning**: "Based on this evidence, I can conclude..."
3. **Action**: "Therefore, I should..."

For example:

1. **Observation**: "I see dark clouds and feel wind picking up"
2. **Reasoning**: "Based on these signs, it's probably going to rain"
3. **Action**: "Therefore, I should bring an umbrella"

This process is grounded in sensory evidence and follows logical reasoning patterns. The conclusion flows naturally from the observation.

Inferential Confusion Process:

1. **Imagined Possibility**: "What if something bad happens?"
2. **Backward Reasoning**: "How could this possibility become real?"
3. **Evidence Creation**: "I can imagine ways this might occur"
4. **Confusion**: "Since I can imagine it, it might be true"

For example:

1. **Imagined Possibility**: "What if I contaminate my family?"
2. **Backward Reasoning**: "How could I become contaminated?"
3. **Evidence Creation**: "I could touch something dirty at the store"
4. **Confusion**: "Since this is possible, I should worry about it"

The key difference is that normal inference starts with evidence and moves toward conclusions, while inferential confusion starts with feared outcomes and works backward to find evidence that could support them.

Research by Aardema and O'Connor published in Cognitive Therapy and Research demonstrates that people with OCD show specific patterns of inferential confusion. They don't have problems with logical reasoning in general - they have problems distinguishing between what they observe and what they imagine.

This distinction is crucial because it changes how we understand what's happening in obsessional thinking. The problem isn't that people with OCD are irrational or illogical. The problem is that they're applying logical reasoning to imagined scenarios as if those scenarios were real.

Maria's grocery store dilemma illustrates this perfectly. Her reasoning isn't flawed - if she actually observed broken items, suspicious behavior, or obvious contamination, her concerns would be completely appropriate. The problem is that she's reasoning about imagined possibilities as if they were observed realities.

The Cognitive Architecture of Obsessional Doubt

To understand how inferential confusion creates obsessional doubt, you need to understand the specific cognitive processes involved. I-CBT theory identifies several key components that work together to generate and maintain doubt:

1. Selective Attention to Possibility People experiencing inferential confusion focus intensely on what *might* happen rather than what *is* happening. They scan their environment not for actual threats, but for potential sources of the threats they're imagining.

Maria walking through the grocery store doesn't notice the normal, safe interactions happening around her. Instead, she focuses on anything that could potentially support her contamination concerns - a person coughing, a spill on the floor, packaging that looks slightly damaged.

2. Imagination Override In normal thinking, sensory evidence trumps imagination. If you see that the stove is off, you don't worry that it might be on just because you can imagine it being on. In inferential confusion, imagination can override sensory evidence.

A person might clearly see that their door is locked but still doubt whether it's really secure because they can imagine ways it might not be properly locked.

3. Categorical Errors People experiencing inferential confusion make systematic errors in how they categorize different types of mental experience. They treat imagined scenarios as if they were observed events, possibilities as if they were probabilities, and hypothetical concerns as if they were real problems.

4. Chain Reasoning Obsessional doubt often involves long chains of "what if" reasoning, where each imagined possibility leads to another, more catastrophic possibility. These chains can extend far beyond any reasonable connection to the original trigger.

Maria's chain might go: "What if I touch something contaminated?" → "What if I bring germs home?" → "What if my children get sick?" → "What if they miss school?" → "What if this affects their education?" → "What if this ruins their future?"

5. Meta-Doubt Perhaps most problematically, people with inferential confusion often doubt their own doubt-resolution processes. They worry not just about specific threats, but about their ability to determine whether threats are real.

"How can I know for sure that I'm not contaminated?" becomes more concerning than the original contamination worry because it suggests that certainty itself might be impossible.

Research published in the Journal of Obsessive-Compulsive and Related Disorders by O'Connor and colleagues shows that these cognitive processes can be measured and modified through specific interventions. This gives us confidence that inferential confusion isn't just a theoretical concept - it's a real, observable phenomenon that can be addressed therapeutically.

Phenomenological Philosophy Meets Cognitive Therapy

I-CBT's theoretical foundation draws heavily from phenomenological philosophy, particularly the work of Edmund Husserl on how people construct their understanding of reality through conscious experience.

Husserl identified several different types of mental acts that people use to engage with their world:

Perception: Direct, sensory-based awareness of present-moment reality **Memory**: Recollection of past experiences **Imagination**: Mental representation of things not currently present **Anticipation**: Expectation of future events **Reflection**: Thinking about thinking

In healthy psychological functioning, people maintain clear distinctions between these different types of mental experience. They know the difference between what they're seeing and what they're imagining, between what they remember and what they're anticipating.

Phenomenological analysis of obsessional thinking reveals that these distinctions become blurred. People experiencing inferential confusion treat imagined scenarios as if they were perceived realities, anticipated problems as if they were current threats, and hypothetical concerns as if they were factual observations.

This philosophical framework provides important insights for understanding why traditional CBT techniques sometimes fall short. If you try to challenge obsessional thoughts using logic and evidence, you're treating them as if they were based on perception and reasoning when they're actually based on imagination being confused with perception.

Traditional CBT approach: "Let's examine the evidence for your contamination concerns." **I-CBT approach**: "Let's look at how your mind created the idea that you might be contaminated."

The first approach treats the obsessional thought as a hypothesis to be tested. The second approach treats it as a product of confused mental processes that need to be clarified.

This distinction matters because people with OCD often have perfectly good reality-testing abilities when they're not caught up in obsessional reasoning. They can evaluate evidence logically and draw reasonable conclusions in most areas of their lives. The problem occurs specifically when imagination gets confused with perception in their area of obsessional concern.

Distrust of the Senses and Over-Reliance on Imagination

One of the most important insights from I-CBT research is that people with OCD often develop what researchers call "distrust of the senses" - a tendency to dismiss or doubt sensory evidence when it conflicts with imagined possibilities.

This creates a paradoxical situation where the more evidence someone has that they're safe, the more they might worry about hidden dangers they can't see.

Consider David, who has checking compulsions around locking his front door. He can see that the door is closed, hear the lock clicking into place, and feel the resistance when he pulls on the door handle. All of his sensory evidence clearly indicates that the door is locked.

But David's imagination suggests possibilities that his senses can't detect: "What if the lock mechanism is broken internally? What if the door looks locked but isn't really secure? What if I think I heard the click but didn't actually turn the key far enough?"

In normal reasoning, clear sensory evidence would resolve these doubts. If you can see, hear, and feel that the door is locked, that's sufficient information to conclude that it's locked.

In obsessional reasoning, sensory evidence becomes suspect specifically because it conflicts with imagined possibilities. The fact that David can't see any evidence of problems with his lock becomes evidence that problems might be hidden from view.

This distrust of sensory evidence is often reinforced by the temporary relief that comes from performing compulsions. When David checks his door multiple times and finally feels "certain" that it's locked, this seems to confirm that his original sensory evidence was insufficient. The compulsion appears to provide more reliable information than simple observation.

Research by O'Connor and Aardema published in Behaviour Research and Therapy demonstrates that this distrust of sensory evidence is learned rather than innate. People with OCD don't have problems with sensory processing in general - they develop specific doubts about sensory evidence in their areas of obsessional concern.

This means that rebuilding trust in sensory evidence can be a key component of treatment. I-CBT includes specific techniques for helping people reconnect with their sensory experience and distinguish between what they observe and what they imagine.

Inverse Inference and Backward Reasoning

One of the most characteristic features of obsessional thinking is what I-CBT researchers call "inverse inference" - the tendency to start with a feared outcome and reason backward to find ways it might be possible.

Normal reasoning follows a forward pattern: **Evidence → Reasoning → Conclusion**

Inverse inference reverses this: **Feared Conclusion → Backward Reasoning → "Evidence"**

This backward reasoning process is particularly problematic because it can find "evidence" for almost any feared outcome, no matter how unlikely.

Let's look at how this works with Anna, who has obsessional concerns about accidentally harming others while driving.

Normal Reasoning About Driving Safety:

- **Observation**: "I'm driving carefully, staying in my lane, following traffic rules"
- **Reasoning**: "Based on my careful driving, the likelihood of an accident is low"
- **Conclusion**: "I can drive safely to my destination"

Anna's Inverse Inference:

- **Feared Outcome**: "What if I hit someone and don't know it?"
- **Backward Reasoning**: "How could this happen without me noticing?"
- **"Evidence" Creation**: "I could have hit someone when I changed lanes, or when I went over that bump, or when I passed that group of pedestrians"
- **Conclusion**: "Since I can imagine ways this could happen, I should check"

The problem with inverse inference is that it makes any feared outcome seem plausible. Once you start with "What if something bad happened?" and work backward, you can always find ways to construct scenarios where the bad outcome is possible.

This leads to what researchers call "possibility proliferation" - the tendency for one imagined possibility to generate multiple related possibilities, each requiring its own consideration and potentially its own compulsive response.

Anna's initial concern about hitting someone while driving can generate dozens of related possibilities:

- "What if I hit someone in the parking lot?"
- "What if I hit someone backing out of my driveway?"
- "What if I hit an animal and it suffered?"

- "What if I clipped a car and didn't notice?"
- "What if someone was hurt because of my bad example of driving?"

Each of these possibilities can then generate its own set of sub-possibilities, creating an endless chain of concerns that have little connection to Anna's actual driving behavior.

Research published in Clinical Psychology Review by Aardema and colleagues shows that inverse inference is maintainted by what they call "imagination inflation" - the tendency for imagined scenarios to become more vivid and compelling through repeated mental rehearsal.

The more Anna imagines hitting someone while driving, the more real and probable this scenario feels to her. This isn't because she has any evidence that she's a dangerous driver - it's because repeated imagination makes unlikely scenarios feel more plausible.

Visual Model: The Complete I-CBT Theoretical Framework

Understanding I-CBT theory requires seeing how all these components fit together into a coherent model of how obsessional thinking develops and maintains itself.

The I-CBT Theoretical Model

TRIGGER SITUATION

(Normal life event)

↓

VULNERABLE SELF-THEME ACTIVATION

(Fear about personal inadequacy)

↓

INVERSE INFERENCE INITIATION

(What if something bad happens?)

↓

IMAGINATION ENGAGEMENT

(Creating possible threat scenarios)

↓

DISTRUST OF SENSES

(Dismissing contradictory evidence)

↓

OBSESSIONAL DOUBT

(Treating possibility as probability)

↓

ANXIETY/DISTRESS

(Emotional response to perceived threat)

↓

COMPULSIVE BEHAVIOR

(Attempt to resolve doubt)

↓

TEMPORARY RELIEF

(Doubt seems resolved)

↓

DOUBT RECURRENCE

(Cycle repeats with next trigger)

This model shows that anxiety and compulsions are not the primary problems in OCD - they're secondary responses to the obsessional doubt created through inferential confusion.

The primary intervention point is the inference process itself - specifically, the moment when someone begins engaging in inverse inference and treating imagined possibilities as if they were realistic concerns.

Let's trace through this model using Maria's grocery store example:

Trigger Situation: Going to grocery store (normal activity)

Vulnerable Self-Theme: "I'm careless and might harm others" (underlying fear about personal adequacy)

Inverse Inference: "What if I cause problems at the store?"

Imagination Engagement: Creating scenarios about breaking things, seeming suspicious, spreading contamination

Distrust of Senses: Dismissing evidence that the store looks normal and safe

Obsessional Doubt: Treating imagined possibilities as realistic concerns requiring attention

Anxiety: Feeling distressed about these perceived threats

Compulsive Behavior: Avoiding the store or engaging in extensive safety behaviors

Temporary Relief: Feeling safer by avoiding the situation

Doubt Recurrence: Next time she needs to go to a store, the cycle repeats

This model suggests that effective treatment should focus on the inference process rather than the anxiety or compulsions. By helping Maria recognize and modify her inverse inference patterns, we can prevent the obsessional doubt from forming in the first place.

Case Analysis: Applying Theory to Clinical Presentations

Let's apply I-CBT theoretical concepts to understand several different OCD presentations:

Case 1: Robert's Contamination Concerns

Robert works in an office and has developed elaborate handwashing rituals. He washes his hands dozens of times per day and avoids touching common surfaces like door handles, elevator buttons, and shared equipment.

Traditional CBT Understanding: Robert has contamination fears that create anxiety. He washes his hands to reduce anxiety. Treatment should use exposure to contaminated items and response prevention of handwashing.

I-CBT Understanding: Robert engages in inverse inference about contamination. He starts with "What if I get contaminated?" and works backward to find evidence for this possibility. His sensory evidence (hands look and feel clean) is dismissed in favor of imagined contamination scenarios. Treatment should focus on his reasoning processes.

Specific I-CBT Analysis:

- **Vulnerable Self-Theme**: "I'm responsible for protecting myself and others from illness"

- **Inverse Inference Pattern**: "What if I picked up germs and don't know it?"

- **Imagination Override**: Creating elaborate contamination stories despite lack of sensory evidence

- **Distrust of Senses**: Dismissing evidence that his hands are clean

- **Possibility Proliferation**: One contamination concern leads to dozens of related worries

Case 2: Jennifer's Checking Behaviors

Jennifer spends forty-five minutes each morning checking appliances before leaving for work. She checks that the coffee maker is off, the stove is off, doors are locked, and windows are closed. Even after checking, she often returns home during lunch to check again.

Traditional CBT Understanding: Jennifer has excessive doubt about safety that creates anxiety. She checks to reduce anxiety about potential disasters. Treatment should focus on reducing checking behaviors and tolerating uncertainty.

I-CBT Understanding: Jennifer engages in inverse inference about household safety. She starts with "What if something bad happens while I'm gone?" and works backward to find evidence for this possibility. Her clear sensory evidence (seeing that appliances are off) is dismissed in favor of imagined disaster scenarios.

Specific I-CBT Analysis:

- **Vulnerable Self-Theme**: "I'm careless and might cause disasters through negligence"
- **Inverse Inference Pattern**: "What if I forgot to turn something off?"
- **Meta-Doubt**: "How can I be sure I really checked properly?"
- **Chain Reasoning**: One safety concern leads to checking every possible hazard
- **Compulsion Reinforcement**: Temporary relief from checking reinforces distrust of initial observations

Case 3: Michael's Pure-O Presentation

Michael experiences intrusive thoughts about harming his infant daughter. He doesn't engage in obvious compulsions but spends hours analyzing his thoughts and seeking reassurance from his wife about whether he's dangerous.

Traditional CBT Understanding: Michael has unwanted intrusive thoughts that create anxiety. He engages in mental compulsions (analyzing thoughts) and reassurance-seeking to reduce anxiety. Treatment should focus on accepting intrusive thoughts without responding to them.

I-CBT Understanding: Michael engages in inverse inference about his potential dangerousness. He starts with "What if I'm dangerous to my daughter?" and works backward to find evidence in his thoughts and behaviors. His clear behavioral evidence (loving, protective parenting) is dismissed in favor of imagined threat scenarios.

Specific I-CBT Analysis:

- **Vulnerable Self-Theme**: "I might be a dangerous person despite appearing normal"

- **Inverse Inference Pattern**: "What if having these thoughts means I'm actually dangerous?"

- **Thought-Action Fusion**: Treating thoughts as equivalent to actions or intentions

- **Mental Compulsions**: Analyzing thoughts to determine their "meaning"

- **Reassurance Seeking**: Attempting to resolve doubt through others' input

The Clinical Implications of I-CBT Theory

Understanding I-CBT theory changes how you approach assessment, case conceptualization, and treatment planning for people with OCD.

Assessment Focus: Rather than focusing primarily on anxiety levels and compulsion frequency, I-CBT assessment explores reasoning patterns, vulnerable self-themes, and the specific ways clients create obsessional doubt.

Case Conceptualization: Instead of viewing OCD as an anxiety disorder maintained by avoidance and compulsions, I-CBT conceptualizes it as a reasoning disorder maintained by inferential confusion and distrust of sensory evidence.

Treatment Planning: Rather than emphasizing exposure and anxiety tolerance, I-CBT treatment focuses on reasoning skills, reality-testing abilities, and reconnection with sensory experience.

This theoretical framework provides a roadmap for understanding why some people develop OCD while others don't, why symptoms persist despite rational knowledge, and why traditional approaches sometimes fall short.

In the next chapter, we'll explore how these theoretical insights translate into practical differences between I-CBT and traditional CBT approaches. You'll see how the same client might be understood and treated differently depending on which theoretical framework guides the intervention.

The power of I-CBT theory lies not just in its ability to explain obsessional thinking, but in its capacity to suggest new and more effective ways of helping people who struggle with doubt, uncertainty, and the endless cycle of "what if" thinking that characterizes OCD.

Understanding the theory is just the beginning. The real test comes in applying these insights to help real people like Maria, Robert, Jennifer, and Michael reclaim their lives from obsessional doubt.

Chapter 4: I-CBT and Traditional CBT Approaches

Dr. Martinez has been treating OCD for fifteen years using exposure and response prevention therapy. She's helped hundreds of clients overcome contamination fears, checking behaviors, and other obsessional symptoms. But lately, she's been frustrated with some of her cases.

"I have clients who complete exposure therapy successfully," she explains to a colleague. "They can touch doorknobs, use public restrooms, leave the house without checking locks. But they still come to sessions talking about doubt. They're functioning better, but they're not really free from the obsessional thinking."

This conversation led Dr. Martinez to explore I-CBT, and what she discovered changed how she understands the difference between managing OCD symptoms and addressing their underlying cause.

The distinction between traditional CBT and I-CBT isn't just academic - it reflects fundamentally different assumptions about what maintains OCD and how change occurs.

Side-by-Side Comparison: Appraisal vs. Inference Models

The easiest way to understand how I-CBT differs from traditional approaches is to compare how each model explains the same clinical presentation.

Case Example: Lisa's Handwashing Compulsions

Lisa washes her hands 30-40 times daily. She knows this is excessive but feels unable to stop. She's particularly concerned about germs from public places, garbage, and her pets.

Traditional CBT Appraisal Model:

Problem Understanding: Lisa has catastrophic thoughts about contamination that create excessive anxiety. She performs handwashing to reduce this anxiety, which reinforces her fear of contamination.

Maintaining Factors:

- Overestimation of threat (believing contamination is more dangerous than it is)
- Overestimation of responsibility (believing she must prevent any possible contamination)
- Intolerance of uncertainty (needing to be 100% sure she's clean)
- Negative appraisals of intrusive thoughts (believing contamination thoughts are significant)

Treatment Approach:

- Cognitive restructuring to challenge catastrophic thoughts
- Exposure to contamination sources with response prevention
- Anxiety management techniques
- Uncertainty tolerance training
- Behavioral experiments to test contamination beliefs

Expected Outcome: Lisa learns that contamination anxiety decreases naturally without handwashing, that most contamination fears are unrealistic, and that she can function normally despite uncertainty about cleanliness.

I-CBT Inference Model:

Problem Understanding: Lisa creates obsessional doubt about contamination through faulty reasoning processes. She treats imagined contamination possibilities as if they were realistic probabilities, leading to doubt that requires resolution through handwashing.

Maintaining Factors:

- Inverse inference (starting with "What if I'm contaminated?" and working backward)
- Distrust of sensory evidence (dismissing clear evidence that she's clean)
- Imagination override (treating imagined contamination as equivalent to observed contamination)
- Categorical errors (confusing possibility with probability)
- Vulnerable self-theme ("I'm careless and might harm others through contamination")

Treatment Approach:

- Reasoning skills training to recognize inverse inference
- Reality-sensing exercises to rebuild trust in sensory evidence
- Distinguishing imagination from perception
- Narrative exercises to create alternative, reality-based stories
- Building confidence in normal reasoning processes

Expected Outcome: Lisa learns to recognize when she's creating obsessional doubt through faulty reasoning, develops skills for staying connected to sensory reality, and stops generating contamination concerns that have no basis in actual evidence.

This comparison reveals several key differences between the approaches:

Different Problem Definitions: Traditional CBT sees Lisa's problem as excessive anxiety about realistic concerns (contamination does exist, but she overestimates the threat). I-CBT sees her problem as generating unrealistic concerns through faulty reasoning (she creates contamination doubt where none should exist).

Different Maintaining Factors: Traditional CBT focuses on how Lisa responds to her intrusive thoughts and anxiety. I-CBT focuses on how Lisa creates the thoughts and doubt in the first place.

Different Treatment Targets: Traditional CBT aims to change Lisa's relationship with contamination anxiety. I-CBT aims to change the reasoning processes that create contamination doubt.

Different Expected Outcomes: Traditional CBT expects Lisa to function better despite continuing to have some contamination thoughts. I-CBT expects Lisa to stop generating unrealistic contamination thoughts altogether.

Research published in Behaviour Research and Therapy by O'Connor and colleagues suggests that these different approaches can lead to different patterns of improvement, with I-CBT showing particular advantages for clients who have difficulty with traditional exposure-based methods.

The Role of Exposure: Why I-CBT Takes a Different Path

One of the most striking differences between I-CBT and traditional CBT is the role of deliberate exposure to feared situations.

Traditional ERP therapy is built on the principle that people with OCD need to face their fears directly in order to learn that their anxiety will decrease naturally without performing compulsions. This requires deliberately exposing people to anxiety-provoking situations and preventing their usual avoidance or safety behaviors.

I-CBT takes a fundamentally different approach. Rather than focusing on anxiety reduction through exposure, I-CBT focuses on reasoning correction through education and skill-building.

Why Traditional ERP Uses Exposure:

Theoretical Basis: Fear conditioning theory suggests that people with OCD have learned to associate neutral stimuli (doorknobs, public restrooms) with danger through classical conditioning. Exposure provides extinction trials that break these learned associations.

Mechanism of Change: Repeated exposure to feared stimuli without negative consequences teaches the brain that these stimuli are actually safe, leading to reduced anxiety over time.

Treatment Process: Clients deliberately seek out increasingly challenging exposure situations while resisting compulsions, gradually building tolerance for anxiety and uncertainty.

Why I-CBT Doesn't Use Deliberate Exposure:

Theoretical Basis: Inference theory suggests that people with OCD generate doubt through faulty reasoning rather than learned fear associations. The problem isn't conditioned anxiety - it's confusion between imagination and reality.

Mechanism of Change: Learning to recognize and correct faulty reasoning processes prevents obsessional doubt from forming, eliminating the need for compulsive responses.

Treatment Process: Clients learn reasoning skills, practice reality-sensing exercises, and develop confidence in their ability to distinguish realistic from unrealistic concerns.

This difference has important practical implications:

Client Experience: ERP requires people to deliberately feel anxious and distressed as part of the treatment process. I-CBT focuses on education and skill-building that can feel less threatening and more empowering.

Treatment Tolerance: Some people find ERP too difficult and drop out of treatment. Research suggests that I-CBT may be more acceptable to clients who struggle with exposure-based approaches.

Generalization: ERP typically requires exposure to each specific feared situation. I-CBT teaches general reasoning skills that can apply to any situation where obsessional doubt might arise.

Let's see how this plays out with Marcus, who has checking compulsions around leaving the house.

Traditional ERP Approach for Marcus:

- Gradual exposure to leaving the house with minimal checking
- Response prevention (not going back to check locks, appliances)
- Building tolerance for uncertainty about home security
- Repeated practice leaving the house despite anxiety
- Learning that anxiety decreases without checking

I-CBT Approach for Marcus:

- Understanding how inverse inference creates doubt about home security
- Learning to distinguish between sensory evidence (seeing that the door is locked) and imagination (what if it's not really secure?)
- Practicing reality-sensing exercises to build confidence in observation
- Creating alternative narratives based on actual evidence
- Developing general skills for recognizing obsessional reasoning

Different Outcomes: After successful ERP, Marcus can leave the house despite feeling some anxiety and uncertainty. After successful I-CBT, Marcus doesn't generate unrealistic doubts about home security in the first place.

Research published in Clinical Psychology Review by Ost and colleagues found that I-CBT can be as effective as ERP for reducing OCD symptoms, with some clients showing preference for the I-CBT approach due to its focus on understanding and skill-building rather than anxiety tolerance.

Treatment Targets: Reasoning vs. Anxiety Management

The different theoretical foundations of traditional CBT and I-CBT lead to different treatment targets and different definitions of successful outcomes.

Traditional CBT Treatment Targets:

Primary Target: Anxiety and distress associated with obsessional thoughts *Secondary Targets*:

- Avoidance behaviors and safety-seeking
- Overestimation of threat and responsibility
- Perfectionism and need for certainty
- Maladaptive coping strategies

Success Criteria:

- Reduced frequency and intensity of compulsions
- Decreased anxiety in previously feared situations
- Improved functioning in work, relationships, and daily activities
- Increased tolerance for uncertainty and anxiety

I-CBT Treatment Targets:

Primary Target: Reasoning processes that create obsessional doubt *Secondary Targets*:

- Distrust of sensory evidence

- Confusion between imagination and perception
- Vulnerable self-themes that trigger inverse inference
- Reliance on compulsions for doubt resolution

Success Criteria:

- Decreased generation of obsessional doubt
- Improved reasoning skills and reality-testing
- Increased confidence in sensory evidence
- Reduced need for compulsions due to lack of doubt

These different targets lead to different therapy experiences:

Traditional CBT Session Focus:

- "How anxious did you feel in that situation?"
- "Were you able to resist the compulsion?"
- "What thoughts went through your mind?"
- "How can we challenge those thoughts?"

I-CBT Session Focus:

- "How did your mind create doubt in that situation?"
- "What reasoning process led to the obsessional thought?"
- "What sensory evidence did you have available?"
- "How can you distinguish what you observed from what you imagined?"

Case example with Patricia, who has contamination concerns about her kitchen:

Traditional CBT Treatment for Patricia: *Week 1-2*: Psychoeducation about OCD and anxiety *Week 3-4*: Cognitive restructuring to challenge contamination thoughts *Week 5-8*: Gradual exposure to kitchen contamination with response prevention *Week 9-12*: Generalization to other contamination situations *Week 13-16*: Relapse prevention and maintenance

Patricia's Experience: Learns to tolerate anxiety about kitchen contamination, can cook and clean normally despite some lingering doubts, develops general anxiety management skills.

I-CBT Treatment for Patricia: *Week 1-2*: Understanding the obsessional sequence and reasoning errors *Week 3-4*: Identifying how inverse inference creates contamination doubt *Week 5-8*: Reality-sensing exercises and building trust in sensory evidence *Week 9-12*: Creating alternative, reality-based narratives about kitchen safety *Week 13-16*: Generalizing reasoning skills to prevent future obsessional doubt

Patricia's Experience: Learns to recognize when she's creating unrealistic contamination concerns, develops confidence in her ability to assess real vs. imagined threats, stops generating contamination doubt in the first place.

Both approaches can lead to significant symptom improvement, but they target different mechanisms and can result in different types of change.

Conceptualizing Intrusive Thoughts Differently

One of the most fundamental differences between traditional CBT and I-CBT lies in how each approach understands intrusive thoughts themselves.

Traditional CBT View of Intrusive Thoughts:

Basic Assumption: Intrusive thoughts are normal mental events that become problematic when people respond to them with excessive concern, self-criticism, or attempts at control.

Treatment Implication: People need to learn to accept intrusive thoughts without fighting them or engaging in compulsions in response to them.

Key Interventions:

- Mindfulness and acceptance of thoughts
- Cognitive defusion (seeing thoughts as mental events rather than facts)
- Response prevention (not acting on thoughts)
- Reducing thought-action fusion (understanding that thoughts don't equal actions)

I-CBT View of Intrusive Thoughts:

Basic Assumption: Many intrusive thoughts in OCD are not random mental events but products of specific reasoning processes that confuse imagination with reality.

Treatment Implication: People can learn to recognize and modify the reasoning processes that create intrusive thoughts, potentially reducing their frequency and intensity.

Key Interventions:

- Understanding how obsessional thoughts are generated
- Distinguishing between realistic concerns and products of inverse inference
- Building skills for reality-testing and sensory grounding
- Preventing the reasoning processes that create intrusive thoughts

This difference has significant practical implications:

Scenario: Tom has repeated thoughts about accidentally hitting someone while driving

Traditional CBT Approach: "These thoughts are just mental noise that your brain produces. Everyone has violent or dangerous thoughts sometimes. The problem isn't having these thoughts - it's how much attention you pay to them and how much they distress you. We need to help you accept these thoughts without fighting them or trying to prove they're not true."

I-CBT Approach: "These thoughts are products of a specific reasoning process where your mind starts with 'What if I hit someone?' and works backward to find evidence that this might have happened. Your brain is treating imagined possibilities as if they were realistic concerns. We can help you recognize when this reasoning process is happening and develop skills for staying connected to what you actually observed while driving."

Different Client Experiences:

Traditional CBT: Tom learns to tolerate having thoughts about hitting people while driving. He accepts that these thoughts will probably continue but develops skills for not responding to them with anxiety or checking behaviors.

I-CBT: Tom learns to recognize when his mind is creating unrealistic concerns about hitting people. He develops confidence in his ability to distinguish between actual driving problems and products of obsessional reasoning.

Research by Aardema and O'Connor published in the Journal of Behavior Therapy and Experimental Psychiatry suggests that this different approach to intrusive thoughts can lead to different patterns of symptom change, with I-CBT showing particular benefits for reducing the frequency and believability of obsessional thoughts themselves.

Higher Tolerability and Acceptability Findings

One of the most important practical differences between I-CBT and traditional CBT approaches relates to treatment tolerability - how easy or difficult clients find the treatment process.

Multiple studies have found that I-CBT may be more acceptable to certain clients than traditional exposure-based approaches. This isn't surprising given the different demands each treatment places on clients.

Traditional ERP Demands:

- Deliberately seeking out anxiety-provoking situations
- Tolerating high levels of distress during exposure exercises
- Resisting strong urges to perform safety behaviors
- Accepting uncertainty and incomplete resolution of fears
- Continuing exposure practice despite temporary increases in anxiety

I-CBT Demands:

- Learning about reasoning processes and how obsessional thoughts form
- Practicing reality-sensing and grounding exercises
- Distinguishing between observation and imagination
- Developing alternative explanations for situations
- Building confidence in normal reasoning abilities

Research published in Psychotherapy and Psychosomatics by O'Connor and colleagues found several advantages for I-CBT in terms of treatment acceptability:

Lower Dropout Rates: Studies suggest that fewer people discontinue I-CBT treatment compared to traditional ERP, possibly because I-CBT doesn't require deliberately increasing anxiety and distress.

Greater Treatment Satisfaction: Clients often report that I-CBT helps them understand why they have OCD symptoms rather than just how to cope with them. This sense of understanding can be empowering and reduce self-criticism.

Reduced Treatment-Related Anxiety: Because I-CBT doesn't require deliberate exposure to feared situations, some clients experience less anticipatory anxiety about therapy sessions themselves.

Better Engagement: The educational focus of I-CBT can appeal to clients who prefer understanding their condition to confronting their fears.

Let's examine specific tolerability differences through Elena's experience with contamination OCD:

Elena's Experience with Traditional ERP: Elena started ERP therapy with high motivation but struggled with the exposure requirements. Her homework assignments included touching public doorknobs without washing her hands, using public restrooms without extensive cleaning rituals, and gradually reducing her shower time from two hours to thirty minutes.

"I understood the logic," Elena explains, "but actually doing the exposures felt overwhelming. I would sit in the parking lot outside public restrooms for twenty minutes trying to work up the courage to go in. Even when I managed to complete an exposure, I felt terrible for hours afterward. I started dreading therapy sessions because I knew we would plan more exposures that would make me feel awful."

Elena completed eight sessions of ERP before discontinuing treatment. While she showed some improvement in her ability to tolerate contamination anxiety, she never felt comfortable with the approach and struggled with homework compliance.

Elena's Experience with I-CBT: Six months later, Elena tried I-CBT with a different therapist. The initial sessions focused on understanding how her mind created contamination doubts through specific reasoning processes.

"Instead of forcing myself to touch contaminated things, we talked about how my brain was generating contamination stories when there was no evidence to support them. I learned about inverse inference and how I was confusing what I imagined might be true with what I could actually observe. This made so much more sense to me."

Elena's I-CBT homework assignments included reality-sensing exercises (paying attention to what she could actually see, hear, and feel), distinguishing between observations and interpretations, and practicing alternative explanations for everyday situations.

"The homework felt like learning new skills rather than torturing myself. I could see how these exercises were building my confidence in my own perceptions rather than just forcing me to endure anxiety."

Elena completed all sixteen sessions of I-CBT and maintained her improvements at six-month follow-up. She reported high satisfaction with the treatment and felt that she understood her OCD in a way that helped prevent symptom recurrence.

Research Findings on Tolerability:

A comprehensive review by Aardema and colleagues published in Clinical Psychology Review found several consistent patterns:

Client Preference: When offered a choice between I-CBT and traditional ERP, approximately 60% of clients chose I-CBT, citing its educational focus and lower anxiety demands.

Completion Rates: I-CBT showed completion rates of 85-90% compared to 70-75% for traditional ERP in most studies.

Treatment Satisfaction: Post-treatment satisfaction ratings were consistently higher for I-CBT, with clients particularly appreciating the focus on understanding rather than enduring.

Therapist Feedback: Therapists reported that I-CBT felt more collaborative and less confrontational than traditional ERP, leading to better therapeutic relationships.

Decision Tree: Choosing Between I-CBT and Traditional CBT

The research on treatment effectiveness and acceptability suggests that both I-CBT and traditional CBT can be effective for treating

OCD, but different approaches may be optimal for different clients and situations.

Here's a practical decision tree for choosing between approaches:

Consider I-CBT as First-Line Treatment When:

- Client has previously dropped out of exposure-based treatment
- Client expresses strong preference for understanding over confronting fears
- Client shows high levels of treatment anxiety or avoidance
- Client has primarily cognitive obsessions with minimal overt compulsions
- Client demonstrates good introspective and reasoning abilities
- Client has comorbid conditions that make exposure therapy challenging

Consider Traditional CBT as First-Line Treatment When:

- Client specifically requests exposure-based treatment
- Client has well-defined behavioral compulsions and clear triggers
- Client shows good tolerance for anxiety and distress
- Client has previously responded well to exposure-based interventions
- Time constraints require brief, intensive treatment
- Therapist has extensive ERP training but limited I-CBT experience

Consider Combined or Sequential Approaches When:

- Client shows partial response to either approach alone

- Different symptoms might benefit from different interventions
- Client is interested in both understanding and confronting their fears
- Severe symptoms require multiple intervention strategies

Red Flags for Either Approach:
- Active psychosis or severe cognitive impairment
- Substance abuse interfering with treatment engagement
- Severe depression requiring immediate intervention
- Safety concerns that require crisis management

Let's see how this decision tree might apply to different cases:

Case 1: Michael - Pure-O Presentation Michael has intrusive thoughts about harming his children but no overt compulsions. He engages in extensive mental reviewing and reassurance-seeking. He's highly intelligent and motivated to understand his condition.

Decision Tree Analysis: Michael's primarily cognitive symptoms, strong preference for understanding, and absence of clear behavioral targets make I-CBT an excellent first-choice option. Traditional ERP would struggle to identify appropriate exposure exercises for his mental obsessions.

Case 2: Sandra - Contamination with Clear Compulsions Sandra has contamination fears with extensive handwashing, cleaning, and avoidance behaviors. She's completed exposure therapy before with partial success and is specifically requesting "the treatment where you touch dirty things" because she believes she needs to confront her fears directly.

Decision Tree Analysis: Sandra's clear behavioral symptoms, previous exposure therapy experience, and specific treatment preference make traditional ERP an appropriate choice, possibly with I-CBT elements added to address any residual cognitive symptoms.

Case 3: David - Treatment-Resistant Checking David has completed two rounds of ERP for checking behaviors with minimal improvement. He becomes extremely anxious during exposure exercises and has difficulty completing homework assignments. He's frustrated with therapy and considering discontinuing treatment.

Decision Tree Analysis: David's poor response to traditional approaches and high treatment anxiety make I-CBT an excellent second-line option. The different mechanism of action might address factors that weren't targeted in his previous treatments.

Clinical Vignettes Comparing Treatment Approaches

To illustrate how these different approaches work in practice, let's follow three clients through both traditional CBT and I-CBT treatments to see how the approaches differ in real clinical situations.

Vignette 1: Rachel's Symmetry and Ordering Compulsions

Background: Rachel spends 2-3 hours daily arranging objects in her home to achieve perfect symmetry and order. Books must be perfectly aligned, clothes hung in specific sequences, and furniture positioned exactly right. She knows this is excessive but feels intense distress when things are "wrong."

Traditional CBT Approach:

- *Assessment Focus*: Severity of distress when items are out of place, time spent on arranging behaviors, specific triggers for ordering compulsions
- *Conceptualization*: Rachel has learned to associate "imperfect" arrangements with anxiety and uses ordering behaviors to reduce this anxiety
- *Treatment*: Gradual exposure to imperfect arrangements with response prevention of correcting behaviors
- *Session 1*: Psychoeducation about OCD and the anxiety-avoidance cycle

- *Session 3*: Begin with minor asymmetries (one book slightly out of place) for 10 minutes
- *Session 6*: Progress to larger disruptions (several books out of order) for 30 minutes
- *Session 10*: Major disruptions (entire bookshelf disorganized) for several hours
- *Outcome*: Rachel learns to tolerate imperfect arrangements despite some continuing discomfort

I-CBT Approach:

- *Assessment Focus*: How Rachel determines that arrangements are "wrong," what makes an arrangement feel "right," reasoning processes behind ordering needs
- *Conceptualization*: Rachel creates doubt about arrangement adequacy through inverse inference and perfectionist reasoning
- *Treatment*: Understanding how the mind creates "wrongness" perceptions and building confidence in "good enough" arrangements
- *Session 1*: Exploring how Rachel decides when something is "wrong" vs. "right"
- *Session 3*: Understanding inverse inference ("What if this arrangement isn't perfect?")
- *Session 6*: Reality-sensing exercises to distinguish actual problems from imagined imperfections
- *Session 10*: Creating flexible standards based on functional rather than perfectionist criteria
- *Outcome*: Rachel stops generating doubt about arrangement adequacy in the first place

Vignette 2: James's Health Anxiety and Body Checking

Background: James checks his body constantly for signs of illness, particularly lumps, changes in moles, or unusual sensations. He spends hours daily examining himself and frequently seeks medical reassurance for minor symptoms.

Traditional CBT Approach:

- *Assessment Focus*: Frequency of body checking, health anxiety levels, medical reassurance-seeking patterns
- *Conceptualization*: James overestimates health threats and uses checking behaviors to reduce anxiety about illness
- *Treatment*: Exposure to health uncertainty with prevention of checking and reassurance-seeking
- *Progress*: Gradual reduction of checking time, tolerating physical sensations without investigation, learning to live with health uncertainty
- *Challenges*: James struggles with exposure exercises and frequently seeks subtle reassurance
- *Outcome*: Reduced checking behaviors but continued underlying health anxiety

I-CBT Approach:

- *Assessment Focus*: How James determines whether physical sensations are "normal" or "concerning," reasoning processes behind health doubts
- *Conceptualization*: James creates health doubts through inverse inference and distrust of normal body sensations
- *Treatment*: Learning to distinguish normal body awareness from obsessional health monitoring

- *Progress*: Understanding how the mind creates health doubts, practicing normal body awareness without scrutiny
- *Advantages*: James finds the educational approach less threatening than deliberate health uncertainty
- *Outcome*: Reduced generation of health doubts and improved confidence in normal body sensations

Vignette 3: Karen's Moral and Religious Scrupulosity

Background: Karen experiences intrusive thoughts about blasphemy and moral transgression. She engages in extensive mental reviewing, confession, and prayer rituals to "undo" perceived sins.

Traditional CBT Approach:

- *Assessment Focus*: Frequency and intensity of moral/religious intrusions, time spent on ritual behaviors, impact on religious practice
- *Conceptualization*: Karen catastrophizes about moral thoughts and uses rituals to reduce anxiety about spiritual consequences
- *Treatment*: Exposure to moral/religious uncertainty with response prevention of ritual behaviors
- *Challenges*: Difficulty creating appropriate exposures for moral concerns, conflict with genuine religious beliefs
- *Limitations*: Hard to distinguish between healthy religious practice and obsessional behavior

I-CBT Approach:

- *Assessment Focus*: How Karen distinguishes between genuine moral concerns and obsessional doubts, reasoning processes behind scrupulosity

- *Conceptualization*: Karen creates moral doubt through inverse inference and confusion between thoughts and actions
- *Treatment*: Understanding difference between realistic moral reflection and obsessional doubt-generation
- *Advantages*: Can work within Karen's religious framework while addressing obsessional reasoning
- *Outcome*: Maintained religious practice while eliminating obsessional doubt about moral status

Integration and Future Directions

The comparison between I-CBT and traditional CBT approaches reveals that both have important contributions to make to OCD treatment. Rather than viewing them as competing approaches, many therapists are beginning to integrate elements of both.

Potential Integration Models:

Sequential Integration: Starting with I-CBT to address reasoning processes, then adding exposure elements for remaining behavioral symptoms

Parallel Integration: Using I-CBT techniques to prepare clients for exposure therapy by improving their reality-testing skills

Symptom-Specific Integration: Using I-CBT for cognitive symptoms and traditional CBT for behavioral symptoms within the same treatment plan

Client-Driven Integration: Allowing clients to choose which elements of each approach feel most helpful and relevant

Research on integrated approaches is still emerging, but early findings suggest that combining elements of both treatments may offer advantages for some clients.

The choice between I-CBT and traditional CBT isn't just a technical decision - it reflects different ways of understanding what OCD is and how change occurs. Traditional approaches focus on changing people's relationship with their symptoms, while I-CBT focuses on changing the processes that create symptoms in the first place.

Both perspectives offer valuable insights, and the future of OCD treatment likely lies in understanding when and how to apply each approach for maximum benefit.

In the next chapter, we'll explore how I-CBT's unique perspective changes our understanding of OCD itself - moving from viewing it as an anxiety disorder to understanding it as a fundamental problem with doubt and reasoning.

Chapter 5: OCD Through the I-CBT Lens

When most people think about OCD, they envision someone washing their hands repeatedly, checking locks obsessively, or arranging objects in perfect order. These visible behaviors capture attention because they seem so obviously excessive and distressing.

But here's what's less obvious: the person engaged in these behaviors isn't primarily struggling with anxiety, fear, or even the behaviors themselves. They're struggling with doubt.

Doubt about whether they're really clean. Doubt about whether the door is actually locked. Doubt about whether the arrangement is truly correct.

This shift from understanding OCD as an anxiety disorder to understanding it as a doubt disorder represents one of the most significant conceptual advances in our field in the past twenty years.

OCD as a Doubt Disorder Rather Than Anxiety Disorder

The traditional view of OCD as an anxiety disorder made intuitive sense. People with OCD look anxious, they report feeling anxious, and their compulsions seem designed to reduce anxiety. For decades, this anxiety-focused understanding guided both research and treatment.

But research by O'Connor and colleagues has revealed something remarkable: when you look closely at what people with OCD actually experience, anxiety is often a secondary response to something more fundamental - obsessional doubt.

The Traditional Anxiety Model of OCD: *Primary Problem*: Excessive anxiety about specific threats *Secondary Problem*:

Compulsive behaviors to reduce anxiety *Mechanism*: Classical conditioning creates learned associations between neutral stimuli and anxiety *Treatment Target*: Reduce anxiety through exposure and habituation

The I-CBT Doubt Model of OCD: *Primary Problem*: Generation of obsessional doubt through faulty reasoning *Secondary Problem*: Compulsive behaviors to resolve doubt *Mechanism*: Inferential confusion creates doubt where none should exist *Treatment Target*: Prevent doubt generation through reasoning correction

This distinction matters because doubt and anxiety are different psychological phenomena that require different interventions.

Anxiety is an emotional response to perceived threat. It's adaptive when the threat is real and problematic when the threat assessment is inaccurate. Anxiety responds well to exposure therapy because repeated contact with feared situations teaches the brain that the threat was overestimated.

Obsessional doubt is a cognitive state where someone cannot achieve certainty about something despite having adequate evidence for a conclusion. It's not based on threat perception but on reasoning processes that treat possibilities as if they were probabilities.

Consider Maria's contamination concerns from earlier chapters. When we explored her experience more carefully, we discovered something important:

"I don't actually feel anxious about germs most of the time," Maria explained. "I feel unsure. Like, I can't tell if I'm contaminated or not. I know it doesn't make logical sense, but I can't shake the feeling that I might be contaminated without knowing it. The anxiety only comes when I try to figure out whether I'm clean or not."

This uncertainty - this inability to feel confident about her cleanliness despite evidence that she's clean - is the core problem. The anxiety is a secondary response to being stuck in this state of unresolvable doubt.

Research published in the Journal of Anxiety Disorders by Aardema and O'Connor found that people with OCD don't actually have higher baseline anxiety levels than control groups. What they have is a specific tendency to generate doubt in their areas of obsessional concern.

Key Differences Between Anxiety and Obsessional Doubt:

Anxiety:

- Emotional response to perceived threat
- Decreases with evidence of safety
- Responds to exposure and habituation
- Can be managed through relaxation and coping skills
- Time-limited (anxiety naturally decreases)

Obsessional Doubt:

- Cognitive state of inability to reach certainty
- Persists despite evidence of safety
- Doesn't respond to exposure alone
- Requires reasoning skills and reality-testing
- Self-perpetuating (doubt feeds on itself)

This explains why some people don't respond well to traditional exposure therapy. If their primary problem is doubt generation rather than anxiety, then learning to tolerate anxiety doesn't address the root cause of their symptoms.

The Vulnerable Self-Theme Concept and Feared Possible Selves

One of I-CBT's most important contributions to understanding OCD is the concept of *vulnerable self-themes* - core fears about personal inadequacy that make people susceptible to obsessional doubt in specific areas.

Unlike general anxiety, obsessional doubt isn't random. It consistently focuses on themes that connect to someone's deepest fears about what kind of person they might be.

Common Vulnerable Self-Themes in OCD:

"I'm a careless person who might cause harm through negligence"

- Leads to checking behaviors, safety concerns, harm obsessions
- Example: "What if I left the stove on and cause a fire?"

"I'm a contaminated person who might spread illness to others"

- Leads to washing behaviors, contamination fears, avoidance
- Example: "What if I picked up germs and make my family sick?"

"I'm a bad person with dangerous impulses"

- Leads to moral scrupulosity, harm obsessions, thought suppression
- Example: "What if having that thought means I'm dangerous?"

"I'm an imperfect person who gets things wrong"

- Leads to perfectionism, ordering behaviors, repetition
- Example: "What if this isn't done exactly right?"

"I'm a dishonest person who might deceive others"

- Leads to confession compulsions, reassurance seeking, self-doubt
- Example: "What if I said something that wasn't completely true?"

These vulnerable self-themes create what I-CBT researchers call "feared possible selves" - nightmare versions of who the person might actually be underneath their conscious intentions and efforts.

The feared possible self isn't just "I might make a mistake" - it's "I might be the kind of person who makes harmful mistakes." It's not just "I might get contaminated" - it's "I might be the kind of person who carelessly spreads contamination to others."

This explains why obsessional concerns feel so threatening and urgent. They're not just about external events - they're about fundamental questions of personal identity and character.

Case Example: David's Checking Behaviors

David spends forty-five minutes each morning checking that all appliances are turned off before leaving for work. He knows this is excessive, but he can't seem to stop.

Surface Level Understanding: David is anxious about house fires and checks appliances to reduce this anxiety.

Vulnerable Self-Theme Analysis: David's obsessional checking connects to a deeper fear that he's a careless, irresponsible person who might cause disasters through negligence. The checking isn't just about preventing fires - it's about proving to himself that he's not the kind of person who would carelessly leave appliances on.

This explains why rational discussions about fire probability don't help David. The issue isn't really about statistical risk - it's about what leaving an appliance on would say about his character and identity.

Understanding Feared Possible Selves:

David's feared possible self might be: "I'm actually a careless, irresponsible person who only appears responsible on the surface. If I don't check carefully, my true negligent nature will be revealed and I'll cause disasters that prove what kind of person I really am."

This feared self feels threatening not because it's likely to be true, but because the consequences of its being true would be catastrophic for David's sense of identity and self-worth.

Obsessional doubt serves as a kind of "test" of these feared possible selves. Each situation that could potentially reveal carelessness becomes a moment where David's true nature might be exposed.

Research by O'Connor and Aardema published in Clinical Psychology Review found that vulnerable self-themes are highly predictive of OCD symptom content and severity. People don't develop obsessions about random topics - they develop obsessions about situations that could potentially confirm their worst fears about themselves.

How Reasoning Errors Create and Maintain Symptoms

Understanding vulnerable self-themes helps explain why people with OCD focus obsessional attention on specific areas, but it doesn't explain how the obsessional thoughts themselves are generated and maintained.

This is where I-CBT's analysis of reasoning errors becomes crucial. People with OCD engage in specific thinking patterns that transform neutral situations into confirmation of their feared possible selves.

The Reasoning Error Sequence:

1. **Trigger Situation**: Normal life event that could theoretically connect to vulnerable self-theme

2. **Vulnerable Self-Theme Activation**: Unconscious fear about personal inadequacy is triggered

3. **Inverse Inference Initiation**: "What if this situation reveals something bad about me?"

4. **Evidence Generation**: Searching for ways the feared outcome could be possible

5. **Imagination Override**: Treating imagined possibilities as if they were observed probabilities

6. **Doubt Creation**: Feeling uncertain about the situation despite lack of evidence for concern

Let's trace this sequence through Jennifer's experience with moral scrupulosity:

Trigger Situation: Jennifer has a brief, unwanted thought about something inappropriate during a religious service.

Vulnerable Self-Theme Activation: "I might be a secretly immoral person who only appears religious on the surface."

Inverse Inference Initiation: "What if having this thought means I'm not really a good person?"

Evidence Generation: "Good people probably don't have thoughts like this. The fact that I had this thought might mean something significant about my true character."

Imagination Override: Treating the possibility that thoughts reveal character as if it were an established fact.

Doubt Creation: "I can't be sure whether I'm actually a good person or just pretending to be good."

This sequence shows how normal mental events (everyone has unwanted thoughts occasionally) get transformed into identity-threatening crises through specific reasoning errors.

Key Reasoning Errors in OCD:

Inverse Inference: Starting with feared outcomes and working backward to find evidence *Category Errors*: Treating thoughts as actions, possibilities as probabilities, imagination as perception *Out-of-Context Reasoning*: Applying information inappropriately to unrelated situations *All-or-Nothing Thinking*: Requiring perfect certainty or complete safety *Thought-Action Fusion*: Believing that thoughts are equivalent to actions or intentions

These reasoning errors are maintained by what researchers call the "inferential confusion cycle":

The Inferential Confusion Cycle:

1. Reasoning error creates obsessional doubt
2. Doubt feels urgent and important
3. Compulsive behavior temporarily reduces doubt
4. Relief confirms that the doubt was "real" and important
5. Next similar situation triggers the same reasoning pattern
6. Cycle repeats and strengthens over time

This cycle explains why OCD symptoms tend to worsen over time without treatment. Each cycle strengthens both the reasoning errors and the person's confidence that their obsessional doubts are meaningful and important.

The Obsessional Narrative and Its Power

One of I-CBT's most important insights is that people with OCD don't just have isolated thoughts - they create elaborate *obsessional narratives* that connect their fears, behaviors, and identity into coherent (but inaccurate) stories about themselves and their world.

These narratives are powerful because they feel complete and explanatory. They provide answers to important questions: Why do I feel this way? What does this mean about me? What should I do about it?

Components of Obsessional Narratives:

Character: The person as someone who might be fundamentally flawed or dangerous *Plot*: How ordinary situations could reveal or trigger this fundamental flaw *Conflict*: The ongoing struggle to prevent the flaw from causing harm *Stakes*: What terrible things might happen if vigilance fails *Resolution*: How compulsive behaviors temporarily resolve the narrative tension

Example: Michael's Harm Obsession Narrative

Character: "I might be a dangerous person who appears normal but has violent impulses."

Plot: "Normal situations might trigger these impulses, and I might act on them without realizing it or remembering it clearly."

Conflict: "I must constantly monitor my thoughts and actions to prevent myself from causing harm."

Stakes: "If I fail to monitor carefully, I might hurt someone and destroy both their life and mine."

Resolution: "By avoiding potentially dangerous situations and analyzing my thoughts carefully, I can prevent disaster and prove I'm not actually dangerous."

This narrative feels compelling because it explains Michael's distressing thoughts and provides a framework for managing them. The problem is that the narrative is based on reasoning errors rather than evidence.

How Obsessional Narratives Maintain Symptoms:

Confirmation Bias: The narrative guides attention toward information that supports it and away from information that contradicts it.

Behavioral Reinforcement: Compulsive behaviors that fit the narrative feel meaningful and important, while behaviors that contradict it feel risky and dangerous.

Identity Integration: The narrative becomes part of how the person understands themselves, making it resistant to change.

Social Validation: Other people's concern about the person's symptoms can inadvertently validate the narrative's importance.

Research published in Behaviour Research and Therapy by O'Connor and colleagues found that obsessional narratives are often more predictive of treatment outcome than symptom severity. People with strong, coherent obsessional narratives tend to have more difficulty with traditional treatments because the narratives provide alternative explanations for therapeutic experiences.

For example, if Michael's treatment involves exposure to situations where he might have harm thoughts, his obsessional narrative can interpret this as: "See, even the therapist thinks I might be dangerous, otherwise why would we need to practice with dangerous situations?"

Flowchart: From Trigger to Compulsion via Inferential Confusion

Understanding how all these components work together - vulnerable self-themes, reasoning errors, obsessional narratives, and doubt generation - requires seeing the complete process from initial trigger to compulsive response.

The Complete I-CBT Process Model:

NEUTRAL TRIGGER SITUATION

(Everyday event)

↓

VULNERABLE SELF-THEME ACTIVATION

(Unconscious fear about personal inadequacy)

↓

OBSESSIONAL NARRATIVE ENGAGEMENT

("This situation could reveal something bad about me")

↓

INVERSE INFERENCE INITIATION

("What if...")

↓

REASONING ERROR APPLICATION

(Category errors, out-of-context reasoning, etc.)

↓

IMAGINATION OVERRIDE

(Treating possibilities as probabilities)

↓

OBSESSIONAL DOUBT CREATION

(Feeling uncertain despite adequate evidence)

↓

ANXIETY/DISTRESS

(Emotional response to identity threat)

↓

COMPULSIVE BEHAVIOR

(Attempt to resolve doubt and protect identity)

↓

TEMPORARY RELIEF

(Doubt seems resolved, identity seems protected)

↓

NARRATIVE REINFORCEMENT

("This proves the threat was real and my response was necessary")

↓

INCREASED VULNERABILITY TO CYCLE REPETITION

(Next trigger more likely to activate the same sequence)

Let's trace this complete cycle through a specific example:

Sarah's Contamination Cycle:

Neutral Trigger: Sarah needs to use a public restroom

Vulnerable Self-Theme: "I might be a careless person who spreads contamination to others"

Narrative Engagement: "Public restrooms are dangerous places where careless people pick up germs and spread them to innocent people"

Inverse Inference: "What if I get contaminated in there?"

Reasoning Errors: Treating the possibility of contamination as a probability, focusing on potential rather than actual contamination sources

Imagination Override: Imagining elaborate contamination scenarios and treating them as realistic concerns

Obsessional Doubt: "I can't be sure whether I'm contaminated or not"

Anxiety: Feeling distressed about potential contamination

Compulsive Behavior: Extensive handwashing and cleaning rituals

Temporary Relief: Feeling "clean" and therefore safe

Narrative Reinforcement: "Good thing I washed carefully, otherwise I might have contaminated my family"

Increased Vulnerability: Next time she needs to use a public restroom, the cycle is more likely to activate

This complete model shows why focusing only on anxiety or compulsions misses the real mechanism driving OCD. The anxiety and compulsions are secondary responses to the doubt created through inferential confusion.

It also shows why traditional exposure therapy sometimes falls short. Even if Sarah learns to use public restrooms without extensive washing, she might continue generating contamination doubt through the same reasoning processes. The behavioral change doesn't address the underlying doubt-creation mechanism.

Multiple Case Examples Across OCD Presentations

To illustrate how the I-CBT understanding applies across different OCD presentations, let's examine several cases that show how the same underlying processes create different symptom patterns.

Case 1: Religious Scrupulosity - Father Thomas

Presentation: Father Thomas experiences intrusive thoughts about blasphemy during religious services and spends hours confessing and performing prayer rituals to "undo" these thoughts.

Vulnerable Self-Theme: "I might be a secretly irreligious person who is deceiving my congregation and God"

Obsessional Narrative: "True priests don't have blasphemous thoughts. Having these thoughts might mean I'm not actually called to religious life and am misleading people about my spiritual state."

Reasoning Errors: Thought-action fusion (treating thoughts as equivalent to beliefs), inverse inference (starting with "What if I'm not truly religious?" and finding evidence), category errors (treating unwanted thoughts as chosen thoughts)

Doubt Generation: "I can't be sure whether I'm truly religious or just going through the motions"

Compulsive Resolution: Confession and prayer rituals that temporarily restore confidence in his religious identity

Case 2: Perfectionism - Dr. Rodriguez

Presentation: Dr. Rodriguez rewrites patient notes dozens of times, checks and rechecks medication calculations, and arrives at work hours early to review her preparations.

Vulnerable Self-Theme: "I might be an incompetent doctor who appears professional but makes dangerous mistakes"

Obsessional Narrative: "Good doctors never make mistakes. Any error I make could harm patients and reveal that I don't deserve to practice medicine."

Reasoning Errors: All-or-nothing thinking (requiring perfect performance), inverse inference ("What if I made a mistake I didn't notice?"), catastrophic thinking (any error could be devastating)

Doubt Generation: "I can't be sure whether my work is actually adequate or just appears adequate"

Compulsive Resolution: Repeated checking and perfecting behaviors that temporarily restore confidence in her competence

Case 3: Relationship OCD - Marcus

Presentation: Marcus constantly analyzes his feelings for his partner, seeks reassurance about their relationship, and worries that he might not truly love her.

Vulnerable Self-Theme: "I might be a selfish person who is incapable of genuine love"

Obsessional Narrative: "People in real love don't have doubts. Having these doubts might mean I'm deceiving both of us and will eventually hurt someone I care about."

Reasoning Errors: Emotional reasoning (treating feelings as facts), inverse inference ("What if I don't really love her?"), perfectionist thinking (expecting constant certainty about emotions)

Doubt Generation: "I can't be sure whether my feelings are genuine or just what I want to believe"

Compulsive Resolution: Reassurance-seeking and relationship analysis that temporarily restore confidence in his feelings

Case 4: Health Anxiety - Patricia

Presentation: Patricia checks her body constantly for signs of illness, researches symptoms online, and seeks frequent medical reassurance.

Vulnerable Self-Theme: "I might be an unhealthy person who misses important health warning signs"

Obsessional Narrative: "Healthy people notice health problems early. If I don't monitor carefully, I might miss something serious and die because of my negligence."

Reasoning Errors: Probability overestimation (treating unlikely health problems as probable), inverse inference ("What if I have a serious illness I haven't noticed?"), catastrophic thinking (any symptom could be dangerous)

Doubt Generation: "I can't be sure whether I'm actually healthy or just not noticing problems"

Compulsive Resolution: Body checking and medical reassurance that temporarily restore confidence in her health

These cases show that while OCD presentations can look very different on the surface, they share the same underlying structure:

- Vulnerable self-themes that create identity threats
- Reasoning errors that generate obsessional doubt
- Compulsive behaviors that temporarily resolve doubt
- Narrative reinforcement that maintains the cycle

Understanding this common structure allows I-CBT to use similar interventions across different OCD presentations, focusing on the reasoning processes rather than the specific content of obsessions.

What This New Understanding Means for Treatment

Viewing OCD as a doubt disorder rather than an anxiety disorder has profound implications for how we approach treatment:

Assessment Changes: Instead of focusing primarily on anxiety levels and compulsion frequency, assessment explores reasoning patterns, vulnerable self-themes, and doubt-generation processes.

Treatment Targets: Rather than anxiety reduction and behavior change, treatment focuses on reasoning correction and doubt prevention.

Intervention Strategies: Instead of exposure and habituation, interventions emphasize education, skill-building, and reality-testing.

Outcome Measures: Rather than symptom reduction alone, success includes improved reasoning abilities and reduced doubt generation.

Relapse Prevention: Instead of anxiety management skills, maintenance focuses on continued application of reasoning skills and early recognition of inferential confusion.

This shift represents more than just a new treatment approach - it's a fundamentally different way of understanding what OCD is and how recovery occurs.

In the next section of this manual, we'll explore how to assess clients from an I-CBT perspective, identifying the specific reasoning patterns and vulnerable self-themes that maintain their symptoms. You'll learn practical tools for understanding how each individual creates obsessional doubt and what interventions will be most effective for addressing their particular pattern of inferential confusion.

The journey from understanding OCD as an anxiety disorder to understanding it as a doubt disorder isn't just theoretical - it opens up entirely new possibilities for helping people reclaim their lives from obsessional thinking.

Chapter 6: The Inference Chain Model and Obsessional Sequences

When Sarah walks into her apartment after work, she notices a small stain on her kitchen counter. Within seconds, her mind launches into a complex sequence that seems almost automatic: *What if that's blood? What if someone broke in and got hurt? What if I touched it and now I'm contaminated? What if I spread disease to my family?* Before she knows it, she's spending two hours scrubbing every surface in her kitchen, her heart racing with anxiety.

This isn't just worry spiraling out of control. This is the inference chain in action - a predictable sequence of reasoning that transforms a neutral observation into an obsessional crisis. Understanding this chain represents one of the most powerful tools in I-CBT, both for therapists learning to identify the pattern and for clients who need to recognize how their minds create suffering from nothing.

The inference chain model reveals something remarkable about OCD: it's not random chaos. It follows a specific, traceable path from trigger to compulsion, and once you can map this path, you can intervene at multiple points along the way. Think of it like being able to see the blueprint of a building that seemed mysterious from the outside. Suddenly, you know where the support beams are, where the weak points lie, and how the whole structure holds together.

The Anatomy of Obsessional Thinking

Most people experience intrusive thoughts. Research by Rachman and de Silva found that over 90% of people have unwanted, strange, or disturbing thoughts pop into their minds. The difference between normal intrusive thoughts and obsessional thoughts isn't the content - it's what happens next. It's the reasoning process that follows.

In normal thinking, when an odd thought appears, we dismiss it quickly. *That's weird,* we might think, and then move on. But in obsessional thinking, that strange thought becomes the starting point for an elaborate reasoning chain that builds doubt upon doubt until the person feels compelled to act.

The inference chain model maps this progression with scientific precision. It shows us that obsessions aren't mysterious forces that appear from nowhere - they're the logical end result of a specific type of faulty reasoning. And because they follow a pattern, they can be interrupted.

Here's what makes this model so different from traditional approaches: instead of focusing on anxiety management or thought stopping, I-CBT targets the reasoning process itself. We're not trying to help people feel less anxious about their obsessions. We're helping them see how those obsessions were constructed in the first place.

The Five-Stage Sequence

Every obsessional episode follows the same basic structure, though the content varies dramatically from person to person. O'Connor and Aardema identified five distinct stages that occur in sequence:

Trigger → Obsessional Doubt → Consequence → Anxiety → Compulsion

Let's break down each stage using Sarah's kitchen counter example:

Stage 1: The Trigger The trigger is always something real and observable. Sarah sees an actual stain on her counter. This isn't imagination - there really is something there. Triggers can be internal (a bodily sensation, a random thought) or external (something you see, hear, or touch). The key point is that triggers, by themselves, are neutral. A stain is just a stain.

Stage 2: Obsessional Doubt This is where the reasoning process goes off track. Instead of making a simple, reality-based inference *(probably spilled coffee)*, the mind generates an obsessional doubt:

What if that's blood? This doubt has a particular quality - it's stated as a possibility but treated as if it needs to be taken seriously. The doubt feels urgent and important, even though it's based on no evidence.

Stage 3: Imagined Consequence Once the doubt takes hold, the mind immediately jumps to catastrophic consequences. *If it's blood, then someone was hurt. If I touch it, I'll be contaminated. If I'm contaminated, I'll spread disease to my family.* Notice how quickly we've moved from a simple stain to life-threatening scenarios. Each consequence builds on the previous one, creating an elaborate story of potential disaster.

Stage 4: Anxiety Response The body responds to these imagined consequences as if they were real threats. Heart rate increases, muscles tense, breathing becomes shallow. This anxiety feels completely justified because, in the person's mind, they're facing genuine danger. The emotional response validates the reasoning chain - *I must be right to worry, or why would I feel so scared?*

Stage 5: Compulsive Response To relieve the anxiety and prevent the imagined catastrophe, the person performs compulsions. Sarah scrubs the counter, then the surrounding areas, then anything she might have touched. The compulsion temporarily reduces anxiety, which reinforces the entire chain. *Good thing I cleaned everything, or something terrible might have happened.*

The Cross-Over Point: Where Reality Becomes Fantasy

The most crucial concept in understanding inference chains is the cross-over point - the exact moment when reasoning shifts from reality-based to imagination-based. This is where normal thinking becomes obsessional thinking.

In Sarah's case, the cross-over happens between seeing the stain (reality) and wondering if it's blood (imagination). She crosses from what she can actually observe to what she's imagining might be possible. Once she crosses this line, everything that follows is built on imagination, not evidence.

Identifying cross-over points is like being a detective investigating a crime scene. You need to trace backward from the anxiety and compulsions to find the exact moment when the person stopped responding to real information and started responding to imagined possibilities.

Consider Michael, who checks his door locks repeatedly. The chain might look like this:

- **Trigger:** Walks past his front door
- **Cross-over point:** *What if I didn't lock it properly?*
- **Consequences:** *Someone could break in, steal everything, hurt my family*
- **Anxiety:** Racing heart, sweating
- **Compulsion:** Checking the lock five times

The cross-over happens when Michael moves from the neutral observation (door exists) to the doubt about his memory and actions (what if I didn't lock it?). Everything after that point is imagination building on imagination.

Mapping Common Inference Patterns

While each person's obsessions feel unique and personal, the underlying inference patterns are surprisingly consistent. Research by the Montreal team identified several common templates that obsessional reasoning tends to follow.

The Contamination Chain *Trigger:* Contact with potentially "dirty" object *Doubt:* "What if this is contaminated?" *Consequences:* "I'll get sick, spread germs, harm others" *Cross-over:* Moving from factual observation to imagined contamination

The Responsibility Chain *Trigger:* Situation where harm could theoretically occur *Doubt:* "What if I'm responsible for preventing this?" *Consequences:* "If I don't act, something terrible will happen and it's my fault" *Cross-over:* Assuming inflated personal responsibility for unlikely events

The Uncertainty Chain *Trigger:* Any situation lacking complete certainty *Doubt:* "What if I can't be sure about this?" *Consequences:* "If I'm not certain, disaster is possible" *Cross-over:* Treating normal uncertainty as unacceptable risk

The Identity Chain *Trigger:* Intrusive thought about acting against personal values *Doubt:* "What if this thought means something about who I am?" *Consequences:* "I might be a terrible person who could do horrible things" *Cross-over:* Interpreting random thoughts as meaningful self-information

Understanding these patterns helps both therapists and clients recognize that obsessions aren't random or mysterious. They follow predictable templates, and once you can see the template, you can begin to interrupt the process.

The Role of Obsessional Reasoning

What drives the progression from trigger to compulsion? The answer lies in what O'Connor called "obsessional reasoning" - a specific style of thinking that prioritizes imagined possibilities over observable evidence.

Normal reasoning works like this: observe evidence, consider most likely explanations, act based on probability. If you see a stain, you think about what usually causes stains (spilled drinks, food, normal household activities) and respond accordingly.

Obsessional reasoning reverses this process: imagine possibility, treat it as if it needs serious consideration, act to prevent imagined consequences. The stain becomes a potential biohazard because *what if it could be blood?* The mere fact that something is possible makes it feel important, regardless of how unlikely it actually is.

This isn't stupidity or irrationality. People with OCD often have above-average intelligence and can think perfectly clearly about topics outside their obsessional themes. It's a specific reasoning error that applies only to their vulnerable areas.

Aardema and O'Connor described obsessional reasoning as operating by different rules than normal thinking:

- Possibility equals probability
- Imagination carries the same weight as evidence
- Remote risks demand immediate action
- Uncertainty equals danger
- Responsibility extends far beyond normal limits

Workshop: Creating Inference Chain Maps

Learning to map inference chains is both an art and a science. It requires careful attention to the sequence of thoughts and the subtle shift from reality to imagination. Here's how to approach this crucial skill:

Step 1: Start with the Compulsion Work backward from the observable behavior. What exactly is the person doing? Washing hands, checking locks, seeking reassurance, avoiding certain places? The compulsion is usually the easiest part to identify because it's visible and repetitive.

Step 2: Identify the Anxiety What emotion or physical sensation drives the compulsive behavior? Anxiety is most common, but some people experience disgust, guilt, or a general sense of "wrongness" that needs to be corrected.

Step 3: Trace the Imagined Consequences What disaster is the person trying to prevent? This often involves following a chain of "what if" scenarios. Start with the immediate fear and work backward to more remote consequences.

Step 4: Find the Core Doubt What fundamental uncertainty or possibility is driving the entire sequence? This is usually expressed as a "what if" question that the person can't answer with complete certainty.

Step 5: Locate the Trigger What real, observable event started the chain? This should be something that actually happened, not something imagined. If you can't identify a concrete trigger, keep probing.

Step 6: Pinpoint the Cross-Over This is the most challenging and important step. Find the exact moment when the person's thinking shifted from responding to evidence to responding to imagination.

Let's practice with Jessica, who spends hours rearranging items in her home:

Working backward:

- **Compulsion:** Rearranging objects until they feel "right"
- **Anxiety:** Intense agitation and sense of incompleteness
- **Consequences:** "If things aren't arranged properly, something bad will happen to my family"
- **Doubt:** "What if the arrangement isn't right? What if it's not symmetric enough?"
- **Trigger:** Noticing that objects on her shelf aren't perfectly aligned
- **Cross-over:** Moving from observable asymmetry to belief that arrangement affects family safety

Practice Cases for Sequence Identification

Case 1: David's Driving Anxiety David pulls over his car three times during a ten-minute drive to check if he hit someone. He becomes convinced he felt a bump and heard a sound that might have been impact with a pedestrian.

Your turn to map the chain: What's the trigger? What's the cross-over point? Where does reality end and imagination begin?

Case 2: Maria's Shower Ritual Maria spends two hours in the shower each morning, washing her hair exactly seven times and her body in a specific sequence. She feels that if she doesn't complete the ritual correctly, her day will be ruined and bad things will happen.

Map this sequence: Identify each stage and pay special attention to how the doubt develops into consequences.

Case 3: Robert's Confession Compulsion Robert repeatedly confesses minor mistakes and perceived moral failings to his spouse, friends, and religious leaders. He once spent ten minutes telling his boss about arriving three minutes late to work.

Trace the inference chain: What triggers these episodes? Where does normal self-reflection become obsessional doubt?

Visual Diagrams of Common Patterns

Understanding inference chains becomes much clearer when you can visualize the process. Imagine a flowchart where each box represents a stage in the sequence, with arrows showing the progression from trigger to compulsion.

The Linear Chain This is the simplest pattern: Trigger → Doubt → Consequence → Anxiety → Compulsion. Each stage leads directly to the next, creating a straight-line progression from observation to action.

The Branching Chain Some obsessional sequences develop multiple branches. A single doubt might lead to several different feared consequences, each requiring its own compulsive response. This creates a tree-like structure with one trigger feeding multiple obsessional concerns.

The Looping Chain In some cases, the compulsive behavior creates new triggers that restart the cycle. Checking the lock once leads to doubt about whether the checking was done properly, which leads to more checking, which creates more doubt. This creates a circular pattern that can continue indefinitely.

The Cascade Chain Complex obsessions often involve multiple chains linked together. Completing one compulsive ritual might provide temporary relief, but then triggers a new sequence of doubt and anxiety about a different concern.

The Therapeutic Value of Chain Mapping

Why spend so much time analyzing the inference chain? Because mapping the sequence transforms a mysterious, overwhelming experience into something concrete and workable. When clients can see their obsessions laid out step by step, several important things happen:

First, they realize their suffering isn't random or uncontrollable. There's a clear pattern with identifiable components. This alone often provides significant relief and hope.

Second, they can begin to see where their reasoning went off track. The cross-over point becomes obvious once it's mapped out clearly. They can literally see the moment when they stopped responding to evidence and started responding to imagination.

Third, they understand that they don't need to challenge every aspect of their obsessions. The most efficient intervention points become clear. Rather than fighting the anxiety or trying to resist compulsions through willpower, they can address the reasoning errors that create the entire sequence.

Finally, mapping chains helps predict and prevent future episodes. Once someone understands their typical pattern, they can recognize the early warning signs and intervene before the sequence builds momentum.

Advanced Chain Analysis

As you become more skilled at mapping inference chains, you'll notice subtle variations and complexities that affect treatment planning. Some chains have false starts, where the person begins to develop an obsessional doubt but then dismisses it before it builds into a full sequence. Others have hidden branches that only become apparent after careful analysis.

Pay attention to what O'Connor called "inference themes" - recurring patterns in how a person's mind constructs obsessional scenarios. Some people consistently overestimate danger, others inflate their personal responsibility, and still others focus on uncertainty and the need for perfect knowledge.

The speed of chain development also varies significantly. Some people experience rapid-fire sequences that progress from trigger to compulsion within seconds. Others develop slow-building chains that unfold over hours or days. Understanding the timing helps determine the most effective intervention strategies.

Integration with Treatment Planning

Inference chain mapping isn't just an academic exercise - it directly informs treatment decisions. Different types of chains require different therapeutic approaches, and the specific characteristics of a person's reasoning patterns determine which I-CBT modules will be most beneficial.

Chains dominated by contamination fears need heavy emphasis on reality sensing and evidence evaluation. Responsibility chains require work on appropriate boundaries and realistic assessment of personal control. Uncertainty chains benefit from tolerance-building exercises and acceptance of normal ambiguity.

The cross-over point analysis also guides intervention timing. Some people need to learn to recognize their triggers earlier in the sequence, while others benefit from interrupting the progression at the doubt stage or before consequences escalate.

Understanding inference chains provides the foundation for everything that follows in I-CBT treatment. Without this conceptual framework, interventions can feel random and disconnected. With clear chain mapping, every therapeutic technique has a specific purpose and target within the client's unique reasoning pattern.

Building Your Chain Mapping Skills

Becoming proficient at inference chain analysis takes practice and patience. Start with clear, simple cases before attempting more complex patterns. Pay attention to the language people use - certain phrases signal different stages in the sequence.

"What if" statements usually mark the transition from trigger to doubt. "If that happens, then" indicates consequence development. "I have to" or "I need to" typically introduces compulsive responses. Learning to recognize these linguistic markers helps you navigate the reasoning sequence more efficiently.

Remember that chain mapping is collaborative work. Clients are the experts on their own experience, and they often provide crucial details that aren't immediately obvious. Your job is to help organize their information into a clear, workable structure that reveals intervention opportunities.

The inference chain model represents one of I-CBT's most significant contributions to understanding OCD. By revealing the step-by-step progression from normal observation to obsessional crisis, it transforms mysterious suffering into understandable patterns that can be systematically addressed.

As you develop expertise in mapping inference chains, you'll find that obsessions lose much of their mysterious power. What once seemed like chaotic, unpredictable mental events become clear sequences with identifiable patterns and intervention points.

This knowledge doesn't just help your clients - it changes how you think about OCD itself. Instead of seeing it as a complex mental illness requiring extensive management, you begin to understand it as a specific reasoning error that can be corrected through targeted intervention.

The next chapter builds on this foundation by examining obsessional doubt itself - the central mechanism that drives the inference chain from trigger to compulsion. Understanding doubt will complete your picture of how obsessional thinking develops and how it can be effectively interrupted.

Chapter 7: Obsessional Doubt - The Cornerstone of I-CBT

Marcus stands in his bathroom, toothbrush in hand, staring at the medicine cabinet. He brushed his teeth thirty seconds ago, but now a familiar feeling creeps in: *Did I actually brush them, or did I just go through the motions? What if I only thought about brushing them? What if my mouth isn't really clean?* The doubt feels urgent, demanding, impossible to dismiss. He brushes again, but the relief lasts only moments before the cycle repeats.

This is obsessional doubt in its purest form - a "what if" that refuses to be answered, a question that generates more questions instead of solutions. Understanding this phenomenon sits at the very heart of I-CBT because obsessional doubt isn't just a symptom of OCD - according to the inference-based model, it's the engine that drives the entire disorder.

Most therapeutic approaches treat doubt as something to be managed, tolerated, or gradually reduced through exposure. I-CBT takes a radically different approach: it helps people recognize that obsessional doubt is fundamentally different from normal uncertainty, and once you understand the difference, the doubt loses its power to control behavior.

The Nature of Normal Doubt

To understand what makes obsessional doubt so problematic, we first need to appreciate how normal doubt functions in healthy mental life. Doubt serves an important purpose - it prevents us from acting on insufficient information and encourages us to gather more evidence when needed.

When you hear an unusual noise in your house at night, normal doubt might make you pause and listen more carefully. *Was that the wind, or should I check the doors?* This doubt is productive. It leads to simple action (looking around, checking obvious explanations) and resolves quickly when you find a reasonable answer (tree branch against window, cat knocking something over).

Normal doubt has several key characteristics that distinguish it from its obsessional counterpart. It's proportional to the situation - bigger decisions generate more doubt, trivial matters generate less. It responds to evidence - when you gather relevant information, the doubt diminishes. It has natural limits - at some point, you accept uncertainty and move forward.

Research by Tallis and his colleagues found that normal doubt follows predictable patterns. People experience it most strongly when facing important decisions with unclear outcomes. They resolve it through information gathering, consultation with others, or simple acceptance that perfect certainty isn't always possible or necessary.

Most importantly, normal doubt doesn't dominate consciousness. It arises when relevant, serves its function, and fades into the background when its purpose is complete. It doesn't demand constant attention or generate elaborate behavioral responses.

The Obsessional Doubt Experience

Obsessional doubt operates by completely different rules. Instead of serving as a helpful information-gathering prompt, it becomes a source of ongoing torment that seems impossible to resolve. The content might sound similar to normal uncertainty, but the experience is qualitatively different.

Take Marcus's tooth-brushing doubt. On the surface, it seems reasonable to want clean teeth. The question "Did I brush thoroughly enough?" could be a normal moment of uncertainty. But obsessional doubt transforms this simple question into an urgent crisis that demands immediate action.

Here's what makes obsessional doubt so distinctive: it doesn't respond to evidence. Marcus can see the wet toothbrush, taste the toothpaste, feel the clean sensation in his mouth, but none of this information reduces the doubt. In fact, gathering evidence sometimes makes the doubt stronger by raising new questions: *But what if the toothpaste wasn't distributed evenly? What if I missed spots? What if going through the motions isn't the same as really cleaning?*

O'Connor described obsessional doubt as having a "void quality" - it creates a sense of emptiness or incompleteness that feels intolerable. Unlike normal uncertainty, which people can live with comfortably, obsessional doubt generates an urgent need for resolution that can't be satisfied through normal problem-solving approaches.

The "What If" That Won't Go Away

The signature characteristic of obsessional doubt is its persistence. Normal doubts get answered and disappear. Obsessional doubts seem to regenerate themselves endlessly, often becoming stronger with each attempt to resolve them.

Consider Jennifer, who doubts whether she locked her car. A normal person might think, *Did I lock the car?* walk back to check, see that it's locked, and forget about it. Jennifer experiences the same initial thought, but checking doesn't end the doubt - it spawns new ones: *Did I check the right car? Did I really look carefully? What if the lock mechanism isn't working properly? What if someone saw me check and knows I'm worried about security?*

This regenerative quality distinguishes obsessional doubt from normal uncertainty. Each attempt to resolve the doubt creates new angles of uncertainty instead of providing closure. The doubt seems to have an intelligence of its own, always staying one step ahead of attempts to pin it down.

Aardema and O'Connor identified several mechanisms that keep obsessional doubt alive:

Doubt about doubt - questioning whether previous checking was done properly **Shifting criteria** - raising the bar for what counts as "enough" certainty **New angle generation** - finding fresh reasons to worry about the same concern **Meta-doubt** - doubting one's ability to judge when something is resolved

These mechanisms create what researchers call the "doubt spiral" - a self-perpetuating cycle where attempts to resolve uncertainty generate more uncertainty instead of less.

How Doubt Persists Despite Contradictory Evidence

One of the most puzzling aspects of obsessional doubt is its immunity to evidence. People with OCD often have abundant proof that their fears are unfounded, yet this evidence doesn't reduce their doubt. This apparent irrationality has led many to conclude that OCD isn't really about reasoning at all.

I-CBT offers a different explanation: obsessional doubt persists because it operates in the realm of imagination rather than evidence. When Marcus doubts whether he brushed his teeth properly, he's not really questioning observable facts - he's worried about imagined possibilities that can't be disproven.

The key insight is that obsessional doubt focuses on what might be true rather than what the evidence suggests is true. Evidence can show that something is highly unlikely, but it can rarely prove that something is impossible. As long as any possibility remains, obsessional doubt can latch onto it and treat it as a serious concern.

This explains why reassurance doesn't work for obsessional doubt. When someone asks, "Are you sure I locked the door?" they're not really asking for information about the door's current state. They're asking for a guarantee that their imagined scenario (unlocked door leading to break-in) won't occur. Since such guarantees are impossible to provide, the doubt remains unsatisfied.

Research by Salkovskis demonstrated this principle clearly. When people with OCD received detailed reassurance about their concerns, their doubt decreased temporarily but returned stronger than before. The reassurance actually reinforced the doubt by suggesting that it was a legitimate concern requiring expert attention.

The Void of Uncertainty vs. The Void of Trust

Understanding why obsessional doubt feels so intolerable requires examining what O'Connor called the "void of uncertainty" versus the "void of trust." These represent two fundamentally different relationships with not knowing.

The void of uncertainty characterizes normal doubt. When healthy people encounter uncertainty, they experience it as a temporary gap in knowledge that can potentially be filled through investigation or accepted through recognition that perfect information isn't always necessary or available.

The void of trust represents the obsessional experience. Instead of seeing uncertainty as a normal part of life, people with obsessional doubt experience it as evidence that something is fundamentally wrong. Not knowing becomes intolerable because it suggests lack of control, inadequate preparation, or failure to prevent potential harm.

This distinction explains why traditional anxiety management techniques often fail with OCD. Teaching someone to "tolerate uncertainty" misses the real issue - they're not struggling with uncertainty itself, but with the meaning they attach to not knowing. The problem isn't that they can't handle ambiguity; it's that they've lost trust in their ability to navigate normal uncertainty effectively.

Sarah illustrates this perfectly. When she sees a stain on her counter, the uncertainty about its origin doesn't feel like normal ambiguity. It feels like a dangerous gap in knowledge that could have serious consequences. The doubt isn't really about the stain - it's about her ability to make reasonable judgments and keep herself safe.

Comparison: Normal vs. Obsessional Doubt Characteristics

The differences between normal and obsessional doubt become clearer when we examine them side by side:

Duration and Intensity Normal doubt is proportional and time-limited. It matches the importance of the situation and resolves within a reasonable timeframe. Obsessional doubt is disproportionate and persistent. Minor situations generate major doubt that can last hours, days, or even years.

Response to Evidence Normal doubt decreases when relevant evidence is gathered. People feel satisfied when they have "enough" information to proceed. Obsessional doubt is evidence-resistant. Gathering information often makes the doubt stronger by revealing new uncertainties or raising questions about the evidence itself.

Behavioral Impact Normal doubt leads to proportional action. People might double-check something important or seek advice on major decisions, but they don't let uncertainty paralyze them. Obsessional doubt drives excessive, repetitive behaviors that often interfere significantly with daily functioning.

Emotional Tone Normal doubt feels manageable, even when uncomfortable. People experience it as part of careful decision-making. Obsessional doubt feels urgent and threatening. It generates anxiety, guilt, or disgust that seems disproportionate to the actual situation.

Resolution Patterns Normal doubt has clear endpoints. People reach conclusions, make decisions, and move forward. Obsessional doubt seems to lack natural stopping points. Each resolution attempt leads to new doubts rather than closure.

Content Focus Normal doubt centers on realistic concerns with reasonable probability. People worry about things that could reasonably happen and have meaningful consequences. Obsessional doubt focuses on remote possibilities or scenarios that are highly unlikely but feel catastrophically important.

Clinical Exercise: Doubt Assessment Techniques

Learning to distinguish obsessional from normal doubt is crucial for effective I-CBT implementation. This assessment skill helps both therapists and clients recognize when doubt has crossed the line from helpful caution to problematic obsession.

The Persistence Test Ask about duration and resistance to resolution. Normal doubt gets answered and stays answered. Obsessional doubt keeps returning despite efforts to resolve it. "How long have you been worried about this specific concern?" "When you checked before, did that put the worry to rest?"

The Proportion Test Examine the relationship between the doubt and its importance. Normal doubt matches significance - big decisions generate more uncertainty than trivial ones. Obsessional doubt often inverts this relationship, creating major anxiety about minor issues. "How important is this concern in the context of your overall life?" "How much time and energy has this worry consumed?"

The Evidence Test Explore how the person responds to contradictory information. Normal doubt decreases when evidence suggests a concern is unfounded. Obsessional doubt persists or intensifies despite contrary evidence. "What evidence do you have that your worry is justified?" "When people tell you not to worry about this, how does that affect your concern?"

The Imagination Test Determine whether the doubt focuses on observable facts or imagined possibilities. Normal doubt deals with realistic unknowns that could be clarified through investigation. Obsessional doubt centers on scenarios that exist primarily in imagination. "Is your worry based on something you can see or measure, or is it about something that might possibly happen?"

The Function Test Assess whether the doubt serves a productive purpose. Normal doubt helps people make better decisions or avoid genuine risks. Obsessional doubt consumes resources without providing benefits. "Has worrying about this helped you in any concrete way?" "What would happen if you simply accepted uncertainty about this issue?"

Self-Reflection: Personal Experiences with Doubt

Understanding obsessional doubt isn't just an intellectual exercise - it requires personal reflection on how doubt functions in your own life. This self-awareness helps therapists relate to their clients' experiences and recognize the subtle differences between helpful and harmful uncertainty.

Think about a recent decision you found difficult. Maybe you debated whether to accept a job offer, move to a new apartment, or end a relationship. How did doubt function in that situation? Did it help you gather important information? Did it prevent you from acting too hastily? At what point did you decide you had enough information to proceed?

Now consider whether you've ever experienced doubt that felt different - more persistent, less responsive to evidence, more emotionally charged than the situation seemed to warrant. Perhaps you repeatedly checked whether you sent an important email, despite seeing it in your sent folder. Maybe you worried excessively about a conversation you had, analyzing every word for hidden meanings.

These personal experiences with problematic doubt help you understand what your clients face, though theirs may be more severe and persistent. The key insight is recognizing that obsessional doubt feels qualitatively different from normal uncertainty, not just stronger or more frequent.

Many therapists find that reflecting on their own relationship with doubt helps them develop empathy for the OCD experience. It also helps them recognize that the goal isn't to eliminate all doubt - it's to restore doubt to its proper function as a helpful information-gathering tool rather than a source of ongoing distress.

The Therapeutic Approach to Obsessional Doubt

Traditional CBT approaches often try to reduce doubt through exposure and response prevention. The logic is that if people can learn to tolerate uncertainty without performing compulsions, the doubt will naturally decrease over time. While this approach can be effective, I-CBT suggests a more direct route.

Instead of trying to tolerate obsessional doubt, I-CBT helps people recognize that obsessional doubt isn't actually doubt at all - it's a reasoning error disguised as legitimate uncertainty. Once someone understands the difference between real doubt and obsessional doubt, they can dismiss the latter without needing to build tolerance for the former.

This approach feels more natural to most clients because it aligns with their intuitive sense that obsessional doubt is different from normal uncertainty. They often say things like, "I know this worry doesn't make sense, but I can't stop thinking about it." I-CBT validates this insight by explaining exactly why the worry doesn't make sense and teaching specific techniques for recognizing and interrupting obsessional reasoning.

The key therapeutic insight is that obsessional doubt thrives on being taken seriously as legitimate uncertainty. When someone treats the doubt as a real question requiring an answer, they unknowingly feed its persistence. Learning to recognize obsessional doubt as a reasoning error rather than a genuine concern removes its power to drive compulsive behavior.

Building Doubt Recognition Skills

Developing the ability to distinguish obsessional from normal doubt requires practice and patience. The difference isn't always immediately obvious, especially when someone has been struggling with OCD for a long time and has lost confidence in their judgment.

Start by teaching clients to notice the emotional tone of their doubt. Normal uncertainty feels manageable and proportional. Obsessional doubt feels urgent, threatening, and disproportionate. The emotional intensity often provides the first clue that doubt has crossed into obsessional territory.

Next, help them examine the behavioral impact of their doubt. Normal uncertainty leads to reasonable investigation and then resolution. Obsessional doubt drives repetitive behaviors that don't actually resolve the underlying concern. If someone finds themselves checking, seeking reassurance, or avoiding situations repeatedly, they're likely dealing with obsessional doubt.

Finally, teach them to assess whether their doubt responds to evidence. Normal uncertainty decreases when relevant information is gathered. Obsessional doubt either ignores evidence or uses it to generate new concerns. If gathering information makes the doubt stronger rather than weaker, it's probably obsessional in nature.

The Broader Implications of Understanding Doubt

Recognizing the nature of obsessional doubt has implications beyond OCD treatment. It helps explain why reassurance doesn't work, why avoidance tends to make problems worse, and why traditional problem-solving approaches often fail with obsessional concerns.

This understanding also helps family members and friends respond more effectively to someone struggling with OCD. Instead of providing endless reassurance or becoming frustrated with "irrational" behavior, they can learn to recognize obsessional doubt and avoid reinforcing it through well-meaning but counterproductive responses.

For therapists, understanding obsessional doubt provides a clear rationale for I-CBT interventions. Instead of trying to reduce anxiety or build distress tolerance, the focus shifts to correcting reasoning errors and restoring healthy doubt function. This approach often feels more efficient and targeted than traditional methods.

Preparing for Intervention

Understanding obsessional doubt sets the stage for effective intervention, but it's important not to rush into trying to eliminate doubt before the client fully grasps its nature. Premature intervention attempts often fail because the person still treats obsessional doubt as legitimate uncertainty that needs to be resolved.

The assessment and education phase around doubt typically takes several sessions, particularly with clients who have longstanding OCD. They may need time to observe their own doubt patterns and begin to recognize the differences between normal and obsessional uncertainty. This foundation work is crucial for successful intervention later in treatment.

Remember that helping someone recognize obsessional doubt isn't about convincing them their concerns are ridiculous or unimportant. It's about helping them see that certain types of doubt function differently than others and require different responses. This nuanced understanding respects their experience while providing tools for change.

The Foundation for Everything That Follows

Mastering the concept of obsessional doubt provides the foundation for all subsequent I-CBT interventions. Without this understanding, techniques like reality sensing and inference chain interruption can feel arbitrary or superficial. With clear comprehension of doubt's role in maintaining obsessions, these interventions make perfect sense as targeted responses to specific reasoning errors.

The next chapter builds on this foundation by examining how primary doubts develop into elaborate secondary inferences that create the catastrophic scenarios driving OCD behavior. Understanding this progression from simple doubt to complex obsessional narrative completes the picture of how reasoning errors create and maintain obsessional suffering.

Chapter 8: Primary and Secondary Inferences in Clinical Practice

When Elena notices her hands feel slightly dry after washing dishes, a simple observation triggers an elaborate mental journey. First comes the primary doubt: *What if the soap didn't clean properly?* Then the mind builds: *If they're not clean, I could spread germs. If I spread germs, my children could get sick. If they get sick, it's because I failed to protect them. If I'm not protecting my children, what kind of mother am I?*

Within thirty seconds, Elena has traveled from slightly dry hands to questioning her fundamental worth as a parent. This progression from simple doubt to catastrophic conclusion illustrates one of I-CBT's most important concepts: the cascade from primary inference to secondary inference, and how this cascade transforms manageable uncertainty into overwhelming crisis.

Understanding this progression is like watching a small spark become a wildfire. The initial doubt might be tiny and manageable, but the secondary inferences that follow can create scenarios so frightening that they seem to justify any amount of compulsive behavior to prevent them.

Understanding the Cascade from Doubt to Catastrophe

The inference cascade follows a predictable pattern that O'Connor and Aardema mapped with scientific precision. It begins with what they called a "primary inference" - the initial doubt that crosses over from reality to imagination. This doubt might seem relatively minor: *What if I didn't lock the door? What if this stain is dangerous? What if I made a mistake?*

But obsessional thinking doesn't stop with primary doubts. Instead, it uses them as building blocks for increasingly elaborate and frightening scenarios. Each "what if" generates another "what if," creating a chain of inferences that leads far from the original concern.

The cascade typically follows this pattern:

- **Primary inference:** Basic doubt about immediate situation
- **Secondary inference 1:** Immediate consequences of the primary doubt
- **Secondary inference 2:** Broader implications of those consequences
- **Secondary inference 3:** Ultimate catastrophic outcomes
- **Meta-inferences:** Doubts about one's ability to handle any of the above

Take Marcus, who doubts whether he turned off his stove. The primary inference is simple: *What if the stove is still on?* But his mind doesn't stop there:

If the stove is on, it could start a fire. If there's a fire, my apartment could burn down. If my apartment burns, the whole building could be destroyed. If the building burns because of my carelessness, people could die. If people die because I was negligent, I'm responsible for their deaths. If I'm capable of such negligence, how can I trust myself with any responsibility?

The progression is remarkable. Within moments, Marcus has moved from a simple appliance concern to questioning his fundamental trustworthiness as a human being. This isn't random catastrophizing - it follows logical connections, but each step moves further from reality and deeper into imagination.

How Secondary Inferences Amplify Primary Doubts

Secondary inferences don't just add to primary doubts - they transform them completely. A manageable uncertainty becomes an urgent crisis because the stakes seem so much higher. The primary doubt about the stove (which could be resolved by a simple check) becomes secondary doubt about personal responsibility for potential deaths (which cannot be resolved through any amount of checking).

This amplification process explains why compulsions often seem so disproportionate to their triggers. When someone spends two hours checking door locks, they're not really responding to uncertainty about the door - they're responding to elaborate scenarios about break-ins, family harm, and personal responsibility that their mind has constructed from a simple doubt about whether they heard the lock click.

Research by the Montreal team found that secondary inferences typically involve three types of escalation:

Magnitude escalation - The consequences become progressively more severe **Scope escalation** - More people become involved in the potential harm **Responsibility escalation** - Personal culpability becomes more extreme

Elena's hand-washing example shows all three types. The magnitude escalates from dry hands to sick children. The scope expands to include family members. The responsibility escalates from simple hygiene to fundamental maternal adequacy.

The Emotional Amplification Process

Each step in the inference cascade doesn't just add logical consequences - it amplifies emotional intensity. The anxiety generated by the primary doubt might be manageable, but the anxiety generated by secondary inferences can feel overwhelming.

This emotional amplification occurs because secondary inferences typically involve themes that are deeply important to the person. Primary doubts might concern practical matters (Is the door locked?), but secondary inferences usually involve core values and fears (Am I a responsible person? Will my family be safe? Am I trustworthy?).

Aardema identified what he called "vulnerable self-themes" - areas where people are particularly sensitive to doubt because they connect to fundamental aspects of identity and values. Common vulnerable themes include:

- **Responsibility and competence** - Am I capable and reliable?
- **Morality and character** - Am I a good person?
- **Safety and protection** - Can I keep myself and others safe?
- **Cleanliness and purity** - Am I acceptable and uncontaminated?
- **Precision and correctness** - Do I do things right?

Secondary inferences tend to converge on these vulnerable themes regardless of where they start. A doubt about hand cleanliness becomes a question about moral character. A concern about door locks becomes uncertainty about protective competence. A worry about making mistakes becomes doubt about fundamental adequacy.

Cognitive Fusion of Inferences

One of the most problematic aspects of the inference cascade is what cognitive scientists call "fusion" - the tendency for all the inferences to feel equally real and urgent. By the time Elena reaches her final concern about maternal adequacy, she's no longer distinguishing between "my hands feel dry" (observable fact) and "I'm a bad mother" (inference based on multiple layers of imagination).

This fusion explains why logical challenges to obsessional thinking often fail. When a therapist points out that dry hands don't actually indicate poor mothering, the client experiences this as missing the point. From their perspective, the connection is obvious and important because all the intermediate steps have become fused into a single, coherent concern.

Cognitive fusion also explains why compulsions provide only temporary relief. Elena might wash her hands until they feel adequately clean, which temporarily reduces anxiety about germs and parenting. But because the underlying inference pattern remains intact, any new trigger can restart the cascade and recreate the same emotional intensity.

Breaking Down Complex Obsessional Stories

Learning to identify and separate primary from secondary inferences is crucial for effective I-CBT intervention. This process requires careful attention to the logical structure of obsessional thinking and the ability to trace backward from final catastrophic concerns to initial triggering doubts.

The key skill is learning to ask the right questions in the right sequence:

"What exactly are you most afraid will happen?" This identifies the final catastrophic scenario that drives the emotional response.

"If that happened, what would it mean about you?" This reveals the vulnerable self-theme underlying the concern.

"What would have to happen for that to occur?" This begins the process of tracing backward through the inference chain.

"And what would have to happen before that?" Continue this process until you reach the primary doubt.

"What actually triggered this whole sequence?" This identifies the real, observable event that started the chain.

Let's apply this process to Robert, who spends hours rewriting emails before sending them:

Final fear: "If I send an email with errors, people will think I'm incompetent and unprofessional."

Vulnerable theme: Competence and professional adequacy

Required conditions: "I'd have to make grammatical mistakes or unclear statements."

Prior conditions: "I'd have to miss errors when proofreading."

Primary doubt: "What if I didn't proofread carefully enough?"

Actual trigger: Feeling uncertain about word choice in one sentence

This analysis reveals that Robert's hours of email revision are driven by a simple uncertainty about word choice that has cascaded into elaborate concerns about professional competence. The primary doubt could be resolved quickly, but the secondary inferences make it feel like a career-threatening crisis.

Detailed Case Study: Following Inference Development

Let's follow the complete inference development in detail using Sarah's contamination concerns from earlier chapters. Understanding her complete cascade illustrates how quickly and dramatically secondary inferences can transform manageable doubts into overwhelming crises.

Initial trigger: Sarah notices a small dark spot on her kitchen counter after work.

Primary inference: "What if that's not just a food stain? What if it's blood or some other contaminant?"

Secondary inference 1: "If it's blood, then someone was injured in my kitchen. If it's another contaminant, it could be dangerous."

Secondary inference 2: "If there was blood from an injury, it could contain diseases. If I touch it, I could become infected."

Secondary inference 3: "If I'm infected, I could spread disease to my family without knowing it."

Secondary inference 4: "If I spread disease to my family, my children could get seriously ill or even die."

Secondary inference 5: "If my children get sick because I brought contamination home, I'm responsible for their suffering."

Meta-inference 1: "If I'm the kind of person who could expose my children to deadly disease through carelessness, what does that say about me as a mother?"

Meta-inference 2: "If I can't even keep my own kitchen safe, how can I trust myself to protect my family in other situations?"

Meta-inference 3: "If I'm questioning my ability to keep my family safe, maybe I'm not fit to be responsible for children at all."

This progression shows how Sarah's two-hour cleaning ritual isn't really about the dark spot on her counter - it's about preventing a scenario where her negligence leads to family illness and reveals her inadequacy as a mother. The primary doubt about stain identity has cascaded into fundamental questions about parental fitness.

Notice how each inference builds logically on the previous one, but also how each step moves further from observable reality. By the end of the sequence, Sarah is responding to elaborate scenarios that exist entirely in imagination, triggered by uncertainty about something that could be resolved with simple observation.

Skills Practice: Identifying Inference Types

Developing the ability to distinguish primary from secondary inferences requires practice with various types of obsessional presentations. Here are several practice cases to help build this crucial skill:

Case 1: James and the Important Phone Call James receives a phone call from his supervisor asking him to "touch base tomorrow about the quarterly report." He spends the rest of the evening convinced he's about to be fired, reviewing every interaction he's had with his boss and preparing explanations for potential failures.

Practice questions:

- What's the primary inference?
- How many secondary inferences can you identify?

- What vulnerable self-theme is involved?
- Where does reality end and imagination begin?

Case 2: Lisa and the Social Media Post Lisa posts a casual comment on social media and then notices it hasn't received any likes or responses after an hour. She begins worrying that she said something offensive, starts analyzing the wording for potential problems, and considers deleting the post.

Analysis task:

- Map the complete inference cascade
- Identify the emotional amplification process
- Determine what makes this obsessional rather than normal social concern

Case 3: David and the Medical Symptom David notices a small headache after a stressful day at work. He begins researching serious neurological conditions online, becomes convinced he might have a brain tumor, and starts planning how to tell his family about his potential terminal diagnosis.

Mapping exercise:

- Trace from trigger to final catastrophic concern
- Identify fusion points where inferences feel equally real
- Determine intervention priorities

The Therapeutic Implications of Cascade Understanding

Understanding inference cascades has profound implications for treatment planning and intervention strategy. Traditional approaches often target final catastrophic concerns or try to reduce overall anxiety levels. I-CBT's cascade analysis suggests more precise intervention points.

The most efficient interventions typically target primary inferences rather than secondary ones. Helping Sarah recognize that her doubt about stain identity is based on imagination rather than evidence is more effective than trying to convince her that maternal adequacy doesn't depend on kitchen cleanliness.

This approach feels more natural to clients because it addresses their concerns at the source rather than asking them to dismiss elaborate scenarios that seem logically connected. Once the primary inference is recognized as unfounded, the entire cascade collapses without requiring separate challenges to each secondary inference.

Timing and Sequence in Cascade Development

Not all inference cascades develop at the same speed or follow identical patterns. Some people experience rapid-fire progressions that move from trigger to catastrophe within seconds. Others develop slow-building cascades that unfold over hours or days, with each inference receiving detailed analysis before progressing to the next level.

Understanding timing is crucial for intervention planning. Rapid cascades require early recognition and immediate intervention techniques. Slow-building cascades allow for more gradual educational approaches that help people observe their own inference development process.

The sequence of secondary inferences also varies between individuals and even between different obsessional themes within the same person. Some people consistently move toward responsibility themes, others toward safety concerns, and still others toward identity and character questions.

Advanced Cascade Analysis

As your skill in cascade analysis develops, you'll begin to notice subtle patterns and variations that affect treatment planning. Some cascades have false branches that the person considers but then dismisses. Others have hidden loops where later inferences circle back to reinforce earlier doubts.

Pay attention to what researchers call "inference density" - how many steps the person's mind takes between trigger and final concern. High-density cascades involve many intermediate steps and tend to be more elaborate and time-consuming to develop. Low-density cascades jump quickly from trigger to catastrophe with fewer intermediate steps.

The emotional trajectory of cascades also varies. Some follow a steady amplification pattern where anxiety increases with each step. Others show emotional plateaus where several inferences develop at similar intensity levels before jumping to a new level of concern.

Integration with Treatment Planning

Cascade analysis directly informs I-CBT module selection and sequencing. Clients with elaborate secondary inference patterns need extensive work on recognizing imagination versus reality. Those with rapid cascade development benefit from early warning system training. People whose cascades consistently target vulnerable self-themes require focused work on those specific identity concerns.

The analysis also reveals which intervention techniques will be most effective. Some cascades are best interrupted early through primary inference challenging. Others benefit from reality sensing techniques that help people recognize when they've moved from evidence to imagination. Still others require work on vulnerable self-themes to reduce the emotional impact of secondary inferences.

Understanding inference cascades provides both therapists and clients with a clear roadmap for recovery. Instead of facing a mysterious and overwhelming disorder, they can see exactly how normal uncertainty gets transformed into obsessional crisis and precisely where to intervene to prevent this transformation.

Building Cascade Interruption Skills

The ultimate goal of cascade analysis is developing the ability to interrupt the progression before it reaches emotionally overwhelming levels. This requires learning to recognize the early warning signs that primary doubt is beginning to generate secondary inferences.

Key warning signals include:

- Rapid escalation of emotional intensity
- Movement from practical concerns to identity questions
- Expansion of consequences beyond immediate situation
- Involvement of other people in catastrophic scenarios
- Shift from "what if" to "what does this mean about me"

Teaching clients to recognize these signals gives them the opportunity to interrupt cascades while they're still manageable rather than waiting until they've developed into full obsessional crises.

The next chapter examines the specific reasoning errors that drive inference cascade development. Understanding these "tricks of OCD" completes the picture of how normal thinking becomes obsessional thinking and provides the foundation for teaching clients to recognize and resist these reasoning traps.

Chapter 9: Reasoning Biases and the Tricks of OCD

Picture OCD as a master con artist who has studied your psychology for years. This con artist knows exactly which buttons to push, which fears to exploit, and which reasoning tricks will convince you that imaginary threats are real emergencies. The con artist is so skilled that even intelligent, rational people fall for the same tricks repeatedly, often while recognizing that the logic "doesn't make sense" but feeling unable to resist it anyway.

This metaphor captures something crucial about obsessional thinking: it doesn't represent random irrationality or general cognitive dysfunction. Instead, it involves specific reasoning errors that follow predictable patterns. Understanding these patterns - what O'Connor called the "reasoning devices" of OCD - transforms mysterious obsessions into recognizable tricks that can be identified and resisted.

The key insight is that people with OCD aren't generally illogical. They often think perfectly clearly about topics outside their obsessional themes. Their reasoning problems are selective, targeting specific areas of vulnerability with surgical precision. Once you can see the tricks being used, they lose much of their power to convince.

Inverse Inference and Backward Reasoning

The most fundamental reasoning error in OCD is what researchers call "inverse inference" - working backward from feared outcomes to present concerns instead of forward from current evidence to logical conclusions.

Normal reasoning follows this pattern: observe current situation → consider likely explanations → draw reasonable conclusions → act accordingly. If you feel tired, you might think about poor sleep, work stress, or coming down with something, then decide whether to rest, take medication, or see a doctor.

Inverse inference reverses this process: imagine feared outcome → work backward to find possible causes → treat those possibilities as current concerns → act to prevent imagined outcome. Instead of reasoning from evidence to conclusion, the person starts with a conclusion (something bad might happen) and works backward to justify worry.

Consider Michael's checking behavior. Normal reasoning would start with observing the door lock's current state and concluding it's secure. Inverse inference starts with the possibility of break-in and works backward: *If someone breaks in, my door would have to be unlocked. If my door could be unlocked, maybe I didn't check it properly. If I might not have checked properly, I should check again.*

This backward reasoning creates what appears to be logical thinking but actually operates independently of evidence. Michael isn't responding to any indication that his door is unlocked - he's responding to the logical possibility that it could be unlocked, given that break-ins are theoretically possible.

Aardema and O'Connor found that inverse inference is particularly powerful because it feels logical to the person using it. The reasoning chain makes sense *if* you accept the initial premise that theoretical possibilities should be treated as practical concerns. The error isn't in the logic itself, but in the starting point.

Category Errors and Misapplied Information

OCD frequently involves what philosophers call "category errors" - applying information or principles from one context to inappropriate situations. This creates reasoning that sounds sensible but misses crucial contextual factors that determine whether the reasoning is actually valid.

A common category error involves applying medical or safety information to everyday situations. Jennifer reads that certain bacteria can survive on surfaces for weeks and concludes that every surface in her home is potentially contaminated. She's not wrong about bacterial survival - the medical information is accurate. But she's making a category error by applying laboratory conditions to her actual living environment.

The same information that's relevant for hospital infection control becomes misleading when applied to normal household cleaning. Jennifer has taken valid data from one category (medical/laboratory) and incorrectly applied it to a different category (everyday/domestic) without adjusting for the different conditions and risk levels.

Another frequent category error involves responsibility standards. People with OCD often apply professional or emergency response standards to personal situations. A person might hold themselves to surgical-level hygiene standards for everyday activities, or demand perfect certainty about decisions that normal people make with incomplete information.

Robert illustrates this pattern with his email checking. He applies error standards appropriate for legal documents or published articles to casual workplace communication. The perfectionist standards aren't wrong in their original context, but they're inappropriately applied to situations that don't require such precision.

Category errors feel convincing because they use genuine information and valid principles. The error lies not in the facts themselves but in failing to recognize when contextual factors make those facts irrelevant or misleading for the current situation.

Irrelevant Associations and Out-of-Context Facts

OCD reasoning often involves connecting genuinely true information to situations where that information isn't relevant. The facts themselves are accurate, but their application to the current concern represents a reasoning error.

Sarah might read that hepatitis can be transmitted through blood contact and then worry about every red stain she encounters. She's not wrong about hepatitis transmission - the medical fact is correct. But she's making an irrelevant association by treating every red stain as potential blood without considering base rates, context, or more likely explanations.

This pattern helps explain why reassurance often backfires with OCD. When someone provides accurate information to address an obsessional concern, they might inadvertently provide new material for irrelevant associations. Telling Sarah that bleach kills viruses might lead her to conclude that everything needs bleach treatment, rather than reducing her worry.

The Montreal team identified several types of irrelevant associations that commonly appear in obsessional reasoning:

Statistical irrelevance - Using accurate statistics from inappropriate populations or contexts **Temporal irrelevance** - Applying past events to current situations despite changed circumstances **Causal irrelevance** - Connecting events that occur together but aren't actually related **Magnitude irrelevance** - Using information about severe cases to evaluate minor situations

David's health anxiety demonstrates statistical irrelevance. He reads that headaches can occasionally indicate brain tumors (true statistic) and applies this to his tension headache after a stressful day (inappropriate context). The medical information is accurate, but the statistical relevance to his specific situation is virtually nil.

Distrust of Senses and Over-Reliance on Possibility

One of OCD's most insidious tricks involves undermining trust in sensory evidence while elevating theoretical possibilities to equal status with observable facts. This creates a reasoning system where imagination carries the same weight as perception.

Normal reasoning prioritizes sensory evidence. If you can see that the door is locked, feel that your hands are clean, or observe that the stove is off, this evidence takes precedence over theoretical concerns about what might possibly be true.

OCD reasoning reverses these priorities. Even clear sensory evidence gets dismissed if theoretical possibilities suggest otherwise. Marcus can see his clean toothbrush, taste the toothpaste, and feel the cleanliness in his mouth, but these sensory inputs get overwhelmed by the possibility that he might have missed something.

This reversal explains why compulsions often provide only temporary relief. The sensory evidence from checking doesn't resolve the underlying doubt because obsessional reasoning has already established that senses can't be trusted. Each checking episode confirms that sensory evidence is inadequate to address the "real" concern, which exists in the realm of possibility rather than perception.

Research by the Montreal team found that this sensory distrust typically develops gradually. People don't suddenly decide their senses are unreliable. Instead, obsessional doubt slowly erodes confidence in perception by repeatedly suggesting that sensory evidence might be insufficient or misleading.

The process often starts with questioning memory rather than immediate perception. "Did I really lock the door?" gradually becomes "Did I look carefully enough when I checked?" which eventually becomes "Can I trust what I'm seeing right now?" This progression explains why checking behaviors often increase over time despite providing repeated confirmation that fears are unfounded.

How OCD Acts as a "Con Artist"

Understanding OCD's reasoning tricks becomes clearer when you think of the disorder as a sophisticated con artist operating within the person's own mind. Like any good con artist, OCD succeeds by exploiting existing vulnerabilities and using the person's own intelligence against them.

The Setup: OCD identifies vulnerable areas - things the person genuinely cares about like family safety, moral character, or personal competence. These aren't arbitrary targets; they're the areas where the person is most motivated to be careful and responsible.

The Hook: OCD presents itself as helping with these important concerns. "I'm just trying to help you be a good parent/responsible person/moral individual." The disorder positions itself as an ally rather than an enemy, making resistance feel dangerous or irresponsible.

The Escalation: Once the person accepts that the concern is legitimate, OCD gradually raises the stakes. What starts as reasonable caution becomes elaborate prevention rituals. The standards for "enough" keep shifting upward, but so gradually that each increase seems justified.

The Payoff: OCD maintains control by providing temporary relief through compulsions. This creates intermittent reinforcement - the most powerful conditioning schedule for maintaining behavior. The person occasionally feels better after checking or cleaning, which confirms that the rituals are "working."

The Cover: When people question the logic, OCD has ready explanations. "Better safe than sorry," "You can never be too careful," "What if you're wrong?" These statements sound reasonable on the surface, making it difficult to argue against them without seeming reckless.

This con artist metaphor helps both therapists and clients understand why intelligence and education don't protect against OCD. Smart people are often better at constructing elaborate justifications for obsessional concerns, making them more vulnerable to sophisticated reasoning tricks rather than less.

Interactive Examples of Each Reasoning Bias

Let's examine how each reasoning error appears in clinical practice through detailed examples that illustrate the specific mechanisms involved.

Inverse Inference Example: Lisa's Social Anxiety Lisa attends a work meeting and notices that one colleague seems quiet and distant. Normal reasoning might consider various explanations: busy day, personal concerns, different personality style. Lisa's inverse inference starts with her fear of social rejection and works backward: *If people dislike me, they would act distant. Tom seems distant. Therefore, he must dislike me. If Tom dislikes me, others probably do too. If others dislike me, my career is in jeopardy.*

The reasoning seems logical, but it starts with an assumed conclusion (social rejection) rather than evaluating evidence about Tom's actual behavior or likely explanations for his demeanor.

Category Error Example: Mark's Home Safety Mark reads a workplace safety manual that emphasizes checking all equipment before use. He begins applying these industrial safety standards to his home, checking every appliance, light switch, and electrical outlet before leaving the house. The safety principles aren't wrong, but they belong to a different category (industrial workplace) with different risk levels and safety requirements than residential settings.

Irrelevant Association Example: Jennifer's Contamination Fears Jennifer learns that antibiotic-resistant bacteria exist in hospitals and concludes that her home requires hospital-level sterilization procedures. She's accurately informed about hospital infections, but she's making irrelevant associations by applying hospital-specific concerns to her home environment, which has completely different bacterial populations and risk factors.

Sensory Distrust Example: Robert's Checking Robert locks his car and begins walking away, but then doubts whether he heard the locking sound clearly. He returns to check, sees the car is locked, but then wonders if he looked carefully enough. He checks again, but then questions whether the lock mechanism might be faulty despite no evidence of problems. Each sensory confirmation gets dismissed by theoretical possibilities that remain unaffected by evidence.

Workshop: Spotting Reasoning Errors in Transcripts

Developing skill in identifying reasoning errors requires practice with real clinical material. Here are excerpted client statements that illustrate different reasoning biases. Try to identify which errors are operating before reading the analysis.

Client Statement 1: "I know statistically the chances are incredibly small, but what if I'm the exception? What if this is the one time something bad happens? I can't take that risk with my family's safety."

Reasoning errors present: This statement shows inverse inference (starting with feared outcome rather than current evidence) and irrelevant association (applying general statistics to specific situation without considering base rates and contextual factors).

Client Statement 2: "I read that professional chefs wash their hands for at least 20 seconds and use specific techniques. If that's what professionals do, shouldn't I be doing the same thing to keep my family safe?"

Analysis: Category error is dominant here - applying professional food service standards to home cooking without considering the different risk levels, contexts, and practical requirements of domestic versus commercial food preparation.

Client Statement 3: "I looked at the stove and it seemed off, but how can I really know? My eyes might have deceived me, or I might not have looked carefully enough. What if I only thought I saw it was off?"

Identify the reasoning errors: This demonstrates sensory distrust and over-reliance on possibility. Clear sensory evidence (seeing the stove off) gets dismissed in favor of theoretical possibilities (might have been deceived) without any evidence that perception is unreliable.

Client Statement 4: "I've been researching this medical condition online, and some people with symptoms like mine ended up having serious diseases. I know most cases are minor, but what if I'm one of the serious ones?"

Practice analysis: Multiple errors appear here: irrelevant association (applying rare case information to common symptoms), inverse inference (starting with feared diagnosis rather than symptom evaluation), and category error (treating internet research as equivalent to medical assessment).

Teaching Clients About Reasoning Errors

Helping clients recognize their own reasoning errors requires careful attention to timing and presentation. People need to understand these concepts intellectually before they can apply them to their own thinking patterns, and they need to feel understood rather than criticized for their reasoning mistakes.

Start by normalizing reasoning errors as common human experiences rather than signs of mental illness or intellectual deficiency. Everyone makes these errors occasionally; OCD simply involves making specific errors more frequently in particular areas of concern.

Use examples from outside the person's obsessional themes to illustrate each concept. This reduces defensiveness and helps them see the patterns more clearly. Once they understand how reasoning errors work in general, they can begin to recognize them in their own thinking.

Emphasize that recognizing reasoning errors isn't about dismissing all concerns or becoming careless. It's about distinguishing between reasonable caution based on evidence and obsessional worry based on imagination. The goal is restoring normal reasoning function, not eliminating appropriate vigilance.

The Cumulative Effect of Multiple Errors

Real obsessional episodes rarely involve just one reasoning error. More commonly, several errors operate simultaneously, creating seemingly airtight justifications for obsessional behavior. Understanding how errors combine helps explain why obsessional reasoning can feel so convincing.

Consider Sarah's contamination episode from earlier chapters. Her reasoning involves:

- **Inverse inference:** Starting with contamination possibility rather than stain observation
- **Category error:** Applying medical/laboratory contamination standards to home environment
- **Irrelevant association:** Connecting household stains to disease transmission
- **Sensory distrust:** Dismissing visual evidence about stain characteristics

When multiple errors operate together, they create mutual reinforcement. Each error provides support for the others, making the overall reasoning seem more solid than any individual component would justify.

Building Error Recognition Skills

Developing the ability to spot reasoning errors in real-time requires practice and patience. Most people need considerable training before they can recognize errors while they're experiencing obsessional episodes rather than only in retrospect.

Start with error identification during calm periods when anxiety levels are low. Review recent obsessional episodes and practice identifying which reasoning errors were involved. This builds familiarity with the patterns without the pressure of real-time recognition.

Gradually work toward recognizing errors during active episodes. This is more challenging because emotional intensity makes clear thinking difficult, but it's ultimately necessary for effective intervention.

Teaching error recognition serves multiple functions beyond simply identifying mistakes. It helps people understand that their obsessional concerns aren't based on careful analysis of real information - they're based on systematic reasoning errors that create false impressions of danger or responsibility.

The Liberation of Understanding

Perhaps the most powerful aspect of learning about reasoning errors is the sense of liberation it provides. People with OCD often feel trapped by concerns that seem simultaneously irrational and compelling. Understanding how reasoning errors create this paradox helps resolve the confusion.

The concerns feel compelling because they're based on sophisticated reasoning that uses real information and logical connections. They feel irrational because the reasoning contains systematic errors that lead to false conclusions. Once people can see the specific errors involved, they no longer need to choose between trusting their intelligence or trusting their intuition that something is wrong.

This understanding provides the foundation for all subsequent I-CBT interventions. Without recognizing reasoning errors, techniques like reality sensing and inference interruption can seem arbitrary or superficial. With clear comprehension of how OCD tricks the mind, these interventions make perfect sense as targeted responses to specific thinking mistakes.

The next chapter examines reality sensing - the process of rebuilding trust in sensory evidence and restoring normal information processing priorities. Understanding reality sensing completes the picture of how to interrupt obsessional reasoning and restore healthy doubt function.

Chapter 10: Reality Sensing and Sensory Information

When Amy stands in her kitchen after washing dishes, she faces a choice that most people never consciously consider. Her eyes tell her the dishes are clean, her hands feel smooth and soap-free, and her nose detects the fresh scent of dish soap. But her mind whispers, *What if you missed something? What if the water wasn't hot enough? What if bacteria are still lurking where you can't see them?*

This moment illustrates the fundamental battle at the heart of OCD: the conflict between sensory evidence and imagined possibilities. In healthy functioning, sensory information carries primary authority in determining what's real and what requires attention. In obsessional thinking, imagination undermines sensory evidence until possibilities feel more compelling than perceptions.

Reality sensing represents I-CBT's approach to restoring normal information processing priorities. It's not about convincing people their fears are irrational - it's about helping them recognize that they already possess reliable tools for distinguishing reality from imagination. The problem isn't that their senses are inadequate; it's that obsessional reasoning has taught them to distrust the very information systems that normally keep thinking grounded in observable truth.

The Primacy of Sensory Evidence in Normal Reasoning

Human beings evolved sophisticated sensory systems for a crucial reason: survival depends on accurate information about current environmental conditions. Our eyes, ears, skin, nose, and taste receptors provide real-time data about what's actually happening around us right now. This information forms the foundation for all adaptive behavior.

Normal reasoning operates on a clear hierarchy of information sources. Direct sensory evidence takes precedence over memory, which takes precedence over imagination. If you can see that the door is locked right now, that trumps memories of past security concerns and imagined scenarios about future break-ins.

This hierarchy isn't arbitrary - it reflects the relative reliability of different information sources. Current sensory input is most accurate because it's happening now under conditions you can observe. Memory becomes less reliable over time and can be influenced by subsequent experiences. Imagination, while valuable for planning and creativity, provides no direct information about current reality.

Research by Gibbon and O'Connor demonstrated this hierarchy in healthy populations. When given conflicting information from different sources, people consistently prioritized current sensory evidence over recalled information or theoretical possibilities. They trusted what they could see, hear, and touch more than what they remembered or imagined.

This prioritization system allows efficient navigation of complex environments. You don't need to research the structural integrity of every chair before sitting down - your senses provide immediate feedback about stability and safety. You don't need to memorize every route through your neighborhood - visual cues guide navigation in real-time.

The system works because it operates automatically, below the level of conscious deliberation. Most of the time, you don't actively decide to trust your senses - you simply respond to sensory information without questioning its reliability or comparing it to imagined alternatives.

How OCD Reverses Information Processing Priorities

Obsessional thinking systematically undermines this natural hierarchy, gradually convincing people that sensory evidence can't be trusted and that imagination provides more reliable guidance for important decisions. This reversal happens so subtly that people often don't recognize it's occurring.

The process typically begins with specific doubts about memory rather than immediate perception. "Did I really lock the door?" seems like a reasonable question after walking away from your car. But when checking confirms the door is locked, obsessional reasoning introduces new doubts: "Did I look carefully enough? Could the lock mechanism be faulty? Might I have been distracted when I checked?"

Each round of checking that fails to provide lasting certainty reinforces the idea that sensory evidence is insufficient for important concerns. The person begins to believe they need more evidence, different evidence, or absolute certainty rather than the "mere" confirmation their senses provide.

Gradually, the doubt spreads from memory to immediate perception. If you can't trust your memory of locking the door, maybe you can't trust your current perception that it's locked either. If your senses missed contamination before, maybe they're missing it now. If you made mistakes in the past, maybe you're making mistakes right now without realizing it.

This progression explains why OCD often gets worse over time despite repeated evidence that fears are unfounded. Each episode of checking or cleaning provides sensory confirmation that the concern was unnecessary, but obsessional reasoning interprets this pattern differently: *If I keep finding that my fears were wrong, maybe I'm not looking hard enough or checking correctly.*

Amy's dish-washing experience illustrates this reversed hierarchy perfectly. Her senses provide clear, immediate evidence that the dishes are clean. But obsessional reasoning has taught her that sensory evidence is unreliable for contamination concerns. Bacteria are invisible, her inspection might be inadequate, and the consequences of missing contamination feel too serious to risk trusting "mere" sensory input.

The reversal becomes complete when imagination begins to feel more reliable than perception. Amy's mental picture of potential bacterial contamination seems more "real" and important than the actual cleanliness she can observe. Her fear-based scenarios about family illness carry more weight than the sensory evidence of successful cleaning.

Inner Senses and Self-Knowledge

Reality sensing involves more than just external sensory information - it also includes what O'Connor called "inner senses" that provide information about internal states, preferences, and knowledge. These inner senses help people recognize what they know, what they want, and what feels right to them personally.

Normal inner sensing allows people to recognize when they've had enough food, when they're tired, when something feels complete, or when a decision aligns with their values. These internal cues guide behavior just as external sensory information guides environmental navigation.

OCD often disrupts inner sensing as thoroughly as it undermines external perception. People lose confidence in their ability to recognize when they've cleaned enough, checked sufficiently, or performed a task adequately. The natural sense of completion gets replaced by anxiety-driven questioning that can continue indefinitely.

Marcus experiences this disruption when brushing his teeth. His inner senses would normally signal when his mouth feels clean and fresh, providing a natural stopping point for the activity. But obsessional doubt overrides these internal cues: *How can you know if it's really clean? What if that feeling of freshness is deceptive? What if you need to brush longer to be truly thorough?*

This disconnection from inner sensing helps explain why people with OCD often seem unable to trust their own judgment about basic activities. They haven't lost the ability to make reasonable assessments - they've learned to distrust the internal cues that would normally guide those assessments.

Restoring inner sensing requires helping people reconnect with their natural capacity to recognize internal states and trust their own knowledge about their experiences. This isn't about building new skills - it's about removing the interference that obsessional reasoning creates with existing capabilities.

The 5-4-3-2-1 Grounding Technique

One of the most practical tools for reality sensing is the 5-4-3-2-1 grounding technique, which systematically engages all five senses to anchor attention in current, observable reality. This technique helps people shift from imagination-based concerns to evidence-based awareness.

The technique involves identifying:

- **5 things you can see** - specific, detailed observations about your visual environment
- **4 things you can touch** - textures, temperatures, pressures you can physically feel
- **3 things you can hear** - sounds present in your current environment
- **2 things you can smell** - any scents or odors detectable right now
- **1 thing you can taste** - flavors currently present in your mouth

The power of this technique lies not just in sensory engagement but in its systematic focus on current, observable information. When Amy uses 5-4-3-2-1 during dish-washing anxiety, she shifts from imagined contamination scenarios to actual sensory data about her current situation.

See: Clean dishes, clear water, organized counter space, normal kitchen lighting, soap bubbles dissipating in the sink

Touch: Smooth dish surfaces, warm water temperature, soft dish towel texture, comfortable counter height

Hear: Water running, dishes clinking gently, normal household sounds, her own breathing

Smell: Fresh dish soap scent, clean water odor, absence of any unpleasant smells

Taste: Normal mouth taste, no unusual flavors, fresh feeling from recent tooth-brushing

This systematic inventory reveals that all available sensory evidence supports cleanliness and normal conditions. The contamination concerns exist entirely in imagination, unsupported by any observable data.

Rebuilding Trust in Perception

Restoring confidence in sensory information requires a gradual process that acknowledges people's learned distrust while systematically demonstrating the reliability of perceptual evidence. This isn't about blind faith in sensation - it's about recognizing that sensory information, while not perfect, provides the best available data about current conditions.

The rebuilding process typically follows several stages:

Stage 1: Recognition of Sensory Distrust Help people recognize how obsessional reasoning has undermined their confidence in perception. This awareness alone often provides significant relief because it explains why they feel torn between "knowing" something logically and feeling unable to trust that knowledge.

Stage 2: Sensory Inventory Practice Systematically practice attending to sensory information in low-anxiety situations. Build familiarity with detailed sensory observation before attempting to apply these skills during obsessional episodes.

Stage 3: Evidence Comparison Compare sensory evidence with obsessional concerns to highlight the distinction between observable facts and imagined possibilities. This isn't about dismissing all concerns, but about recognizing which concerns are supported by current evidence.

Stage 4: Graduated Trust Building Start with less emotionally charged situations and gradually work toward applying sensory trust in more anxiety-provoking circumstances. Success in easier situations builds confidence for more challenging applications.

Stage 5: Integration with Daily Life Incorporate reality sensing into routine activities until it becomes automatic rather than requiring conscious effort.

Robert's email checking provides a clear example of this progression. Initially, he distrusts his perception of what he's written, requiring multiple re-readings to feel confident about content. Through reality sensing work, he learns to trust his initial reading and his internal sense of when communication is clear and appropriate.

Practical Exercises in Reality Sensing

Developing reality sensing skills requires hands-on practice with specific exercises designed to strengthen confidence in perceptual information. These exercises should be practiced regularly, starting in calm situations before applying them during obsessional episodes.

Exercise 1: Detailed Sensory Description Choose an everyday object and spend five minutes describing it using all available senses. Focus on specific, observable details rather than interpretations or concerns. For example, describe a coffee mug by its weight, temperature, texture, color variations, sounds it makes when tapped, any residual tastes or smells.

This exercise builds familiarity with detailed sensory attention and demonstrates how much information the senses actually provide when given focused attention.

Exercise 2: Reality vs. Imagination Sorting When experiencing obsessional concerns, create two lists: "What I can actually observe" and "What I'm imagining might be true." Be specific and detailed in both lists. This exercise clarifies the distinction between evidence-based and imagination-based concerns.

Amy might list: *Observable:* Dishes feel smooth, water runs clear, no visible residue, fresh soap scent, normal kitchen appearance *Imagined:* Invisible bacteria, inadequate cleaning, potential illness, family contamination

Exercise 3: Prediction Testing Use sensory evidence to make predictions about what will happen, then observe outcomes to build confidence in perceptual accuracy. If the dishes look and feel clean, predict that they will remain clean and cause no problems. Track these predictions over time to demonstrate sensory reliability.

Exercise 4: Mindful Daily Activities Practice complete sensory attention during routine activities like showering, cooking, or organizing. Focus entirely on what you can observe through the senses rather than thinking about past performance or future concerns.

Exercise 5: Sensory Anchoring During anxiety-provoking situations, systematically anchor attention in sensory evidence before making decisions about whether action is needed. This prevents imagination from overwhelming perception during emotionally intense moments.

Case Examples: Successful Sensory Rehabilitation

Understanding how reality sensing works in practice becomes clearer through detailed case examples that show the progression from sensory distrust to renewed confidence in perceptual information.

Case 1: Jennifer's Hand-Washing Recovery Jennifer spent up to an hour washing her hands, never feeling confident they were truly clean. Through reality sensing work, she learned to trust specific sensory indicators: smooth skin texture, absence of visible contamination, clean water running off her hands, fresh soap scent, and normal skin appearance.

Initially, she needed to consciously inventory these sensory cues after washing. Gradually, she developed automatic trust in this evidence and could conclude hand-washing based on sensory information rather than anxiety levels. Her washing time decreased to normal duration because she could recognize when the task was actually complete.

Case 2: David's Driving Confidence David repeatedly pulled over to check whether he had hit pedestrians, despite no sensory evidence of impact. Reality sensing helped him trust his senses while driving: he had felt no impact, heard no collision sounds, seen no pedestrians in his path, and observed normal traffic flow continuing around him.

Learning to trust this sensory evidence allowed him to continue driving when obsessional doubts arose. He developed the ability to distinguish between actual sensory information suggesting problems (which would warrant stopping) and imagined possibilities unsupported by evidence (which could be dismissed).

Case 3: Lisa's Social Reality Lisa constantly worried that people disliked her despite no behavioral evidence supporting this concern. Reality sensing helped her attend to actual social cues: genuine smiles, engaged conversation, voluntary interaction initiation by others, and inclusion in group activities.

By focusing on observable social evidence rather than imagined negative judgments, she developed more accurate assessments of her relationships and reduced her need for constant reassurance-seeking.

The Relationship Between Reality Sensing and Anxiety

An important aspect of reality sensing involves understanding the relationship between anxiety and perception. Many people assume that if they feel anxious, there must be something wrong that their senses are missing. I-CBT helps clarify that anxiety can be triggered by imagination independently of sensory evidence.

Normal anxiety responses are triggered by sensory detection of actual threats - seeing danger, hearing alarm signals, feeling physical problems. Obsessional anxiety often operates independently of sensory input, triggered instead by imagined scenarios that aren't supported by current perceptual evidence.

This distinction helps people understand why anxiety reduction techniques alone don't resolve OCD. The anxiety isn't necessarily responding to real environmental threats that need to be addressed - it's responding to imagined possibilities that don't require action.

Reality sensing provides an alternative to using anxiety levels as indicators of danger. Instead of asking "Do I feel worried about this?" people learn to ask "What do my senses tell me about the current situation?" This shift from emotion-based to evidence-based assessment often provides more accurate guidance for appropriate action.

Integration with Other I-CBT Techniques

Reality sensing doesn't operate in isolation - it integrates with other I-CBT techniques to provide comprehensive reasoning rehabilitation. Understanding how these techniques work together helps maximize therapeutic effectiveness.

With Inference Chain Analysis: Reality sensing helps identify the cross-over point where thinking shifts from evidence to imagination. When people can clearly distinguish sensory evidence from imagined possibilities, they can recognize exactly where their reasoning goes off track.

With Doubt Assessment: Reality sensing provides tools for distinguishing realistic from obsessional doubt. Realistic doubts typically involve questions about observable situations that can be resolved through sensory investigation. Obsessional doubts persist despite sensory evidence and focus on imagined possibilities.

With Reasoning Error Recognition: Reality sensing demonstrates how reasoning errors operate by showing the contrast between evidence-based and imagination-based thinking. When people can clearly see what their senses reveal, reasoning errors become more obvious.

Advanced Reality Sensing Applications

As people develop basic reality sensing skills, they can begin applying these techniques to more complex situations and subtle forms of sensory distrust. Advanced applications involve recognizing how obsessional reasoning can corrupt even detailed sensory attention.

Some people develop elaborate checking rituals that appear to involve careful sensory observation but actually represent anxiety-driven repetition rather than genuine information gathering. They might look at the same lock dozens of times without actually processing the visual information because anxiety interferes with attention.

Advanced reality sensing helps distinguish between genuine sensory attention and anxiety-driven pseudochecking. Real sensory attention provides clear information that can guide decision-making. Pseudochecking generates temporary anxiety relief without providing useful information about actual conditions.

Learning this distinction helps people recognize when they're truly gathering information versus when they're performing compulsive rituals disguised as careful observation.

Building Confidence in Sensory Judgment

The ultimate goal of reality sensing work is rebuilding confidence in one's natural capacity for sensory judgment. This isn't about developing new abilities - it's about removing the interference that obsessional reasoning creates with existing perceptual capabilities.

Most people with OCD retain excellent sensory function. Their eyes work fine, their hearing is normal, and their touch sensitivity is intact. The problem isn't with sensory organs but with trust in sensory information. Reality sensing helps restore appropriate confidence in perceptual evidence.

This restoration process requires patience because sensory distrust often develops over years of obsessional thinking. People need time to practice using sensory evidence and observe that it provides reliable guidance for daily decisions.

Success in reality sensing creates positive feedback loops that strengthen confidence over time. When people trust sensory evidence and find that it guides them appropriately, they become more willing to rely on perceptual information in the future.

The Liberation of Trusting Your Senses

Perhaps the most profound benefit of reality sensing work is the sense of liberation it provides. People with OCD often feel trapped in endless cycles of checking and uncertainty because they've lost trust in their natural capacity to assess situations accurately.

Reconnecting with sensory evidence provides a way out of this trap. Instead of relying on anxiety levels, repetitive checking, or other people's reassurance, they can use their own perceptual capabilities to determine when situations are actually safe or tasks are truly complete.

This liberation extends beyond specific obsessional concerns to general life confidence. When people trust their senses again, they feel more capable of navigating daily challenges independently and making reasonable decisions about all kinds of situations.

Reality sensing represents both a specific technique and a fundamental shift in how people relate to information about their world. It restores the natural hierarchy that prioritizes current evidence over past concerns and future possibilities, allowing people to respond to what's actually happening rather than what they imagine might occur.

Integration with Treatment Goals

Reality sensing serves multiple functions within the broader I-CBT framework. It provides immediate tools for managing obsessional episodes, but it also supports long-term recovery by rebuilding fundamental trust in one's own judgment capabilities.

The technique works synergistically with other I-CBT interventions. Inference chain analysis helps people understand how their reasoning goes off track, while reality sensing provides tools for staying on track. Doubt assessment helps distinguish realistic from obsessional concerns, while reality sensing provides methods for resolving realistic doubts appropriately.

Understanding reality sensing completes the foundational knowledge needed for effective I-CBT implementation. The next section of this book will focus on assessment and case formulation, showing how to apply these theoretical concepts to individual clients and specific obsessional presentations.

The journey from sensory distrust to sensory confidence represents one of the most empowering aspects of I-CBT recovery. When people reclaim their natural ability to trust their senses, they regain a fundamental tool for distinguishing reality from imagination - a capability that supports not just OCD recovery but overall psychological well-being and life effectiveness.

Chapter 11: Clinical Assessment in I-CBT

Dr. Martinez sits across from Elena, a 32-year-old marketing professional who describes spending three hours each morning in elaborate cleaning rituals before leaving for work. As Elena recounts her daily struggles, Dr. Martinez listens not just for symptoms, but for something more specific: the reasoning patterns that transform normal hygiene concerns into obsessional crises.

"I know it sounds crazy," Elena says, "but what if the soap didn't actually clean my hands? What if there are still germs that could make my family sick?" This single statement reveals layers of inference-based thinking that traditional assessment might miss entirely. Elena isn't just experiencing anxiety about contamination - she's demonstrating the specific reasoning errors that I-CBT targets for intervention.

Effective I-CBT assessment requires a fundamentally different approach than traditional OCD evaluation. While standard protocols focus primarily on symptom severity and functional impairment, I-CBT assessment examines the underlying reasoning processes that generate and maintain obsessional thinking. This shift from symptom mapping to reasoning analysis provides the foundation for precise, targeted intervention.

The assessment process serves multiple functions beyond simple diagnosis. It educates clients about their own thinking patterns, builds therapeutic rapport through collaborative exploration, and identifies the specific reasoning vulnerabilities that will guide treatment planning. Most importantly, it begins the therapeutic process by helping people recognize the difference between evidence-based and imagination-based thinking.

The Inferential Confusion Questionnaire-Expanded Version (ICQ-EV)

The ICQ-EV represents the cornerstone of I-CBT assessment, specifically designed to measure the reasoning processes that underlie obsessional thinking. Unlike traditional OCD measures that focus on symptom frequency and distress, the ICQ-EV assesses the degree to which people rely on imagination rather than evidence when making important decisions.

Developed by Aardema and O'Connor through extensive research with both clinical and non-clinical populations, the ICQ-EV consists of 30 items that examine different aspects of inferential confusion. Each item presents a scenario that requires choosing between evidence-based and possibility-based reasoning.

Sample items illustrate the questionnaire's focus on reasoning patterns rather than specific symptoms:

"I sometimes think that if something is possible, then it is probable" measures the tendency to treat theoretical possibilities as practical concerns.

"I find myself believing things about situations that I have no evidence for" assesses direct reliance on imagination over observation.

"I trust my hunches about situations more than what I can actually observe" examines the hierarchy of information sources in decision-making.

The questionnaire uses a 6-point Likert scale ranging from "completely disagree" to "completely agree," allowing for nuanced assessment of reasoning tendencies. Scores above 20 typically indicate clinically significant inferential confusion, while scores above 25 suggest severe reasoning difficulties that require intensive intervention.

Research by Wu and colleagues demonstrated strong psychometric properties for the ICQ-EV, with excellent internal consistency and good test-retest reliability. More importantly, the measure showed strong predictive validity for I-CBT treatment response, with higher baseline scores predicting greater benefit from inference-based interventions.

The ICQ-EV provides several advantages over traditional OCD assessment tools. First, it identifies reasoning patterns that remain consistent across different obsessional themes. Someone might score high on inferential confusion regardless of whether their obsessions focus on contamination, harm, or responsibility. Second, it predicts treatment appropriateness more accurately than symptom-based measures. Third, it provides specific targets for intervention by identifying which reasoning errors are most prominent for each individual.

Administering the ICQ-EV requires careful attention to context and explanation. Many clients find some items confusing initially because they're not accustomed to thinking about their thinking processes explicitly. The therapist should frame the questionnaire as an exploration of reasoning styles rather than a test of mental health, emphasizing that different reasoning approaches work better for different situations.

Comprehensive Assessment Protocol: Sessions 1-2

I-CBT assessment typically spans two sessions, allowing sufficient time for thorough exploration of reasoning patterns without overwhelming clients with lengthy evaluation procedures. This extended timeline also permits the therapeutic relationship to develop while gathering assessment information.

Session 1: Initial Exploration and Symptom Mapping

The first session begins with standard clinical interview procedures but quickly shifts toward reasoning-focused inquiry. After establishing basic demographic information and presenting concerns, the assessment explores how obsessional episodes develop from trigger to compulsion.

The therapist should gather detailed examples of recent obsessional episodes, paying particular attention to:

- The specific trigger that initiated the sequence
- The initial doubt or concern that arose
- How that doubt developed into more elaborate concerns
- The reasoning process that connected initial doubt to final catastrophic scenarios
- The evidence available at each stage of the reasoning chain
- The cross-over point where thinking shifted from evidence to imagination

This exploration often requires gentle guidance because clients may not initially recognize the distinction between evidence-based and imagination-based thinking. They might describe elaborate contamination scenarios as if they were realistic concerns rather than imagination-based possibilities.

Elena's assessment illustrates this process. She describes seeing a small stain on her kitchen counter and immediately thinking, "What if that's blood from someone who was injured?" The therapist explores this reasoning: "What evidence did you have that it was blood? What made that possibility feel important enough to worry about? How did you move from seeing a stain to thinking about injury?"

This exploration reveals Elena's reasoning pattern: she treats remote possibilities as serious concerns, relies on imagination rather than observation to assess situations, and applies medical contamination standards to normal household conditions.

Session 1 also includes administration of the ICQ-EV and other relevant questionnaires, with brief discussion of items that the client finds confusing or particularly relevant to their experience.

Session 2: Reasoning Pattern Analysis and Treatment Planning

The second session focuses on analyzing the reasoning patterns identified in session 1 and beginning to help the client recognize these patterns. This session is more educational than the first, introducing basic I-CBT concepts while continuing assessment.

The therapist reviews the ICQ-EV results with the client, highlighting specific reasoning tendencies that emerged from the questionnaire. This discussion should be collaborative and non-judgmental, framing reasoning errors as understandable responses to uncertainty rather than signs of mental illness.

Session 2 also involves detailed exploration of the client's vulnerable self-themes - the core identity areas where obsessional doubt tends to concentrate. Common themes include competence, morality, responsibility, safety, and purity. Understanding these themes helps predict which situations will trigger obsessional episodes and which reasoning errors are most likely to occur.

The session concludes with initial treatment planning discussions, including whether I-CBT appears appropriate for the client's presentation and what modifications might be necessary for their specific reasoning patterns and life circumstances.

Y-BOCS and Supplementary Measures

While the ICQ-EV provides the core I-CBT assessment information, supplementary measures help establish baseline symptom severity and track treatment progress. The Yale-Brown Obsessive Compulsive Scale remains the gold standard for measuring OCD symptom severity and continues to play an important role in I-CBT assessment.

The Y-BOCS provides several types of information that complement ICQ-EV findings:

- Objective symptom severity ratings for comparison with other treatments
- Detailed symptom checklist that helps identify all relevant obsessional themes

- Functional impairment assessment that guides treatment prioritization
- Baseline scores for measuring treatment progress

However, Y-BOCS interpretation requires modification within the I-CBT framework. Traditional interpretation focuses on symptom reduction as the primary treatment goal. I-CBT interpretation emphasizes changes in reasoning patterns, with symptom reduction expected to follow from reasoning improvements.

Research by O'Connor and colleagues found that I-CBT often produces different Y-BOCS improvement patterns than traditional CBT. Instead of gradual symptom reduction across all areas, I-CBT sometimes produces rapid improvement in specific obsessional themes while other symptoms remain temporarily stable. This pattern reflects the reasoning-focused approach that targets underlying mechanisms rather than surface symptoms.

Additional supplementary measures provide important contextual information:

Beck Depression Inventory-II (BDI-II) assesses comorbid depression that might affect treatment response or require concurrent intervention.

Beck Anxiety Inventory (BAI) measures general anxiety levels that can interfere with reasoning-focused work.

Obsessive Beliefs Questionnaire (OBQ) examines cognitive beliefs that often accompany obsessional thinking, such as inflated responsibility, perfectionism, and intolerance of uncertainty.

Dimensional Obsessive-Compulsive Scale (DOCS) provides dimensional assessment of OCD symptoms that complements the Y-BOCS categorical approach.

The key principle in supplementary assessment is using measures that enhance understanding of reasoning patterns rather than simply documenting symptom presence. Each measure should contribute specific information that guides I-CBT treatment planning.

Identifying Suitable Candidates for I-CBT

Not all clients with OCD benefit equally from I-CBT approaches. Research has identified several characteristics that predict positive response to inference-based treatment, allowing therapists to make informed decisions about treatment selection.

Strong Predictors of I-CBT Success:

High ICQ-EV scores indicate significant inferential confusion that responds well to reasoning-focused intervention. Clients who rely heavily on imagination rather than evidence show dramatic improvement when they learn to recognize and correct these reasoning errors.

Preserved insight into the unreasonableness of obsessional concerns suggests intact reality testing that can be strengthened through I-CBT techniques. Clients who know their fears "don't make sense" but feel unable to resist them often benefit significantly from understanding why their reasoning feels so compelling.

Intellectual curiosity about their own thinking processes facilitates engagement with I-CBT's educational approach. Clients who find it interesting to examine their reasoning patterns tend to master the concepts more quickly and apply them more consistently.

Frustration with compulsive behaviors rather than fear of symptom reduction indicates readiness for change-focused intervention. Clients who want to stop their rituals but feel unable to resist them respond well to techniques that address the reasoning driving those behaviors.

Moderate Predictors:

Higher education levels correlate with I-CBT success, possibly because the approach requires understanding abstract concepts about reasoning and inference. However, education level is less important than intellectual curiosity and insight.

Shorter illness duration predicts better outcomes, likely because reasoning patterns haven't become as deeply entrenched. However, I-CBT can benefit people with chronic OCD when other factors are favorable.

Specific obsessional themes show different response rates, with contamination and responsibility concerns typically responding better than symmetry or "just right" feelings that may have stronger biological components.

Characteristics Suggesting Caution:

Very low ICQ-EV scores might indicate that obsessional symptoms aren't primarily driven by inferential confusion. These clients might benefit more from traditional CBT approaches that target different mechanisms.

Significant overvalued ideation where clients truly believe their obsessional concerns are realistic makes reasoning-focused work more challenging. These cases require careful assessment to determine if reality testing is sufficiently intact for I-CBT methods.

Severe comorbid conditions such as psychosis, severe depression, or active substance abuse typically require stabilization before I-CBT can be effectively implemented.

Very poor insight into the unreasonableness of obsessional concerns suggests that reality testing problems might be too severe for reasoning-focused intervention without preliminary work.

Assessing Reasoning Patterns and Vulnerable Themes

Understanding each client's specific reasoning patterns and vulnerable self-themes provides the foundation for individualized treatment planning. This assessment requires careful exploration of how obsessional thinking develops and what core concerns drive the emotional intensity of symptoms.

Reasoning Pattern Assessment:

The assessment should identify which of the common reasoning errors are most prominent for each client. Different people show different patterns, and treatment efficiency improves when interventions target the most active reasoning biases.

Inverse inference assessment involves exploring whether the client typically starts with feared outcomes and works backward to current concerns, or begins with current evidence and reasons forward to logical conclusions.

Category error assessment examines whether the client applies information or standards from inappropriate contexts to their current situations.

Irrelevant association assessment looks for patterns of connecting accurate information to situations where that information isn't relevant.

Sensory distrust assessment evaluates how much confidence the client places in current perceptual evidence versus imagined possibilities.

Marcus provides a clear example of reasoning pattern assessment. His door-checking behavior demonstrates inverse inference (starting with break-in possibility rather than lock evidence), sensory distrust (dismissing visual and tactile evidence of security), and category error (applying high-security standards to normal residential situations).

Vulnerable Theme Assessment:

Vulnerable self-themes represent the core identity areas where obsessional doubt tends to concentrate. These themes are deeply personal and often connect to the client's most important values and relationships.

Common vulnerable themes include:

Competence and adequacy - "Am I capable and reliable enough to handle important responsibilities?"

Moral character - "Am I a good person who can be trusted not to cause harm?"

Safety and protection - "Can I keep myself and loved ones safe from danger?"

Cleanliness and acceptability - "Am I clean and pure enough to be acceptable to others?"

Precision and correctness - "Do I do things carefully and accurately enough?"

Elena's vulnerable theme centers on maternal competence and family protection. Her contamination fears aren't really about germs - they're about whether she's a good enough mother to protect her children from harm. This understanding guides treatment toward addressing competence doubts rather than simply reducing contamination anxiety.

Theme assessment requires gentle exploration because these areas are often emotionally sensitive. The therapist should frame the discussion as understanding what matters most to the client rather than identifying psychological weaknesses.

Sample Assessment Interview with Annotations

The following excerpt from Elena's assessment interview illustrates how reasoning-focused inquiry differs from traditional symptom exploration:

Therapist: "You mentioned spending about three hours on cleaning each morning. Can you walk me through what happened yesterday when you were getting ready for work?"

Elena: "Well, I was washing dishes after breakfast, and I noticed this small dark spot on one of the plates. I couldn't tell what it was."

Therapist: [*Note: Identifying the concrete trigger*] "So you saw an actual spot on the plate. What went through your mind when you noticed it?"

Elena: "I immediately thought, what if that's not just food? What if it's something dangerous, like blood or bacteria that could make my family sick?"

Therapist: [*Note: Cross-over from evidence to imagination*] "So you moved from seeing a spot to wondering if it might be blood or bacteria. What evidence did you have that it was either of those things?"

Elena: "Well, I didn't really have evidence. But I read that hepatitis can survive on surfaces, and my kids use those plates."

Therapist: [*Note: Irrelevant association - medical information applied to household context*] "That's interesting. The hepatitis information is medically accurate, but how likely do you think it was that hepatitis was actually on your breakfast plate?"

Elena: "When you put it that way, probably not very likely. But what if I was wrong? What if this was the one time something dangerous was there?"

Therapist: [*Note: Possibility treated as probability*] "So even though it's unlikely, the possibility feels important enough to take seriously. What did you do with the plate?"

Elena: "I washed it again, but then I started worrying about the other dishes, and the sink, and basically everything in the kitchen."

Therapist: [*Note: Inference cascade from single doubt to elaborate concerns*] "The worry spread from one plate to the whole kitchen. What was going through your mind as that was happening?"

Elena: "I kept thinking, if there was contamination on one thing, it could have spread to everything else. And if I didn't clean it all properly, my kids could get seriously sick. What kind of mother would I be if I let that happen?"

Therapist: [*Note: Vulnerable self-theme - maternal competence*] "So this connected to questions about being a good mother. The spot on the plate somehow became about your adequacy as a parent?"

Elena: "I know it sounds ridiculous when you say it like that, but in the moment, it felt completely logical and important."

This brief exchange reveals Elena's reasoning pattern: inverse inference starting with contamination possibility, irrelevant association connecting medical information to household situations, and cascade development ending in maternal competence concerns. This analysis provides specific targets for I-CBT intervention.

Forms and Questionnaires for Clinical Use

Effective I-CBT assessment requires standardized forms that capture reasoning patterns and track treatment progress. The following assessment package provides necessary evaluation tools:

Primary Assessment Instruments:

- Inferential Confusion Questionnaire-Expanded Version (ICQ-EV)
- Yale-Brown Obsessive Compulsive Scale (Y-BOCS)
- Obsessional Sequence Mapping Worksheet
- Vulnerable Self-Theme Assessment Form

Supplementary Measures:

- Beck Depression Inventory-II (BDI-II)
- Beck Anxiety Inventory (BAI)
- Obsessive Beliefs Questionnaire (OBQ)
- Reality Sensing Self-Assessment

Progress Monitoring Tools:

- Weekly ICQ-EV Brief Version
- Obsessional Episode Tracking Form
- Treatment Progress Rating Scale

- Homework Completion Log

The Obsessional Sequence Mapping Worksheet provides structured exploration of how specific episodes develop from trigger to compulsion. This form guides both assessment and ongoing case conceptualization by helping clients and therapists identify patterns across different situations.

The Vulnerable Self-Theme Assessment Form systematically explores core identity areas where obsessional doubt concentrates. This assessment helps predict which situations will trigger episodes and which reasoning errors are most likely to occur in different contexts.

Progress monitoring forms track changes in reasoning patterns rather than just symptom reduction. The Weekly ICQ-EV Brief Version provides session-by-session assessment of inferential confusion levels, allowing therapists to adjust treatment focus based on reasoning improvements.

Integration with Treatment Planning

Assessment information directly informs treatment planning decisions, including module selection, intervention sequencing, and modification of standard protocols for individual needs. The assessment data should answer several key questions:

Which reasoning errors are most prominent? This determines which I-CBT modules receive emphasis and which cognitive techniques will be most beneficial.

What vulnerable themes drive emotional intensity? This guides how to address the identity concerns that make obsessional doubt feel so compelling.

How quickly do inference chains develop? This affects the timing and intensity of intervention techniques.

What triggers consistently activate obsessional thinking? This helps predict challenging situations and plan preventive strategies.

How much insight does the client have into reasoning errors? This determines the pace of psychoeducation and the complexity of concepts that can be introduced.

Elena's assessment reveals prominent inverse inference and irrelevant association errors, with maternal competence as the primary vulnerable theme. Her inference chains develop moderately quickly (minutes rather than seconds), and she shows good insight into the unreasonableness of her concerns. This profile suggests she'll benefit from standard I-CBT modules with extra emphasis on evidence evaluation and reality sensing techniques.

Cultural and Diversity Considerations

I-CBT assessment must account for cultural differences in reasoning styles, family expectations, and religious or spiritual beliefs that might influence how people think about uncertainty, responsibility, and contamination. What appears to be reasoning errors in one cultural context might represent adaptive thinking in another.

The assessment should explore:

- Cultural or religious beliefs about cleanliness, safety, and responsibility
- Family expectations about perfectionism or protective behaviors
- Language differences that might affect reasoning pattern expression
- Socioeconomic factors that influence risk assessment and prevention behaviors
- Previous trauma or discrimination that might affect trust in institutions or safety assessments

These factors don't contraindicate I-CBT treatment, but they do require modifications in how concepts are presented and which examples are used to illustrate reasoning principles.

Preparing for Treatment

The assessment phase concludes with collaborative treatment planning that builds on the reasoning analysis conducted during evaluation. Clients should leave the assessment sessions with:

- Clear understanding of how their specific reasoning patterns create obsessional episodes //
- Recognition that their symptoms result from correctable thinking errors rather than mysterious mental illness
- Realistic expectations about treatment duration and the types of changes they can expect
- Motivation for engaging in reasoning-focused work rather than symptom management approaches

The assessment phase sets the foundation for everything that follows in I-CBT treatment. By focusing on reasoning patterns rather than symptom catalogs, it provides both therapist and client with a clear roadmap for recovery based on correcting specific thinking errors rather than managing chronic mental illness.

Chapter 12: Case Conceptualization Using the I-CBT Framework

Sarah sits in Dr. Chen's office six weeks into I-CBT treatment, finally understanding why traditional therapy never quite worked for her contamination fears. "I see it now," she says, looking at the case formulation diagram they've been developing together. "I wasn't really worried about germs - I was worried about being the kind of mother who fails to protect her children. The germs were just the story my mind told to justify that deeper fear."

This moment of insight illustrates the power of I-CBT case conceptualization. Unlike traditional formulations that focus on symptom patterns and behavioral chains, I-CBT conceptualization maps the reasoning processes that transform normal protective instincts into obsessional crises. It reveals how vulnerable self-themes interact with reasoning errors to create elaborate obsessional narratives that feel completely compelling yet rest on foundations of imagination rather than evidence.

Case conceptualization in I-CBT serves multiple therapeutic functions. It provides a collaborative framework for understanding symptom development, identifies specific intervention targets, and helps both therapist and client see how seemingly random obsessions actually follow predictable patterns. Most importantly, it transforms the client's relationship with their symptoms from helpless victim to informed analyst of their own thinking processes.

Building a Complete Clinical Picture

I-CBT case conceptualization begins with comprehensive mapping of the client's reasoning profile across multiple domains. This process goes beyond traditional symptom assessment to examine the underlying cognitive architecture that generates obsessional thinking.

The complete clinical picture includes several interconnected components that work together to maintain obsessional patterns:

Triggering Situations and Contexts These represent the real-world circumstances that activate obsessional reasoning. Triggers can be external (seeing stains, hearing news stories, encountering certain situations) or internal (bodily sensations, random thoughts, emotional states). The key is identifying patterns in what consistently activates inference chains.

Sarah's triggers include kitchen activities, bathroom visits, contact with potentially "contaminated" surfaces, and media reports about illness outbreaks. But more specifically, her triggers activate when she's in maternal role situations where family protection feels salient.

Primary Inference Patterns These are the initial reasoning errors that transform neutral triggers into obsessional concerns. Different clients show consistent patterns in how they move from observation to doubt, and understanding these patterns helps predict and prevent future episodes.

Sarah consistently demonstrates inverse inference, starting with contamination possibilities rather than evidence about actual conditions. She also shows irrelevant association, connecting medical information to household situations without considering contextual differences.

Vulnerable Self-Theme Architecture This represents the core identity concerns that give obsessional thinking its emotional power. Vulnerable themes aren't just abstract concepts - they connect to the client's deepest values, most important relationships, and fundamental sense of self.

Sarah's primary vulnerable theme centers on maternal competence and family protection. Her obsessions aren't really about contamination - they're about whether she's adequate as a mother and capable of keeping her children safe from harm.

Inference Chain Development Patterns These show how primary doubts develop into elaborate secondary inferences that create catastrophic scenarios. Understanding chain development helps identify intervention points and predict how thoughts will escalate if left unchecked.

Sarah's chains follow a consistent pattern: environmental trigger → contamination possibility → family exposure risk → child illness potential → maternal failure implications → fundamental inadequacy questions.

Compulsive Response Systems These represent the behavioral and mental strategies the client uses to manage obsessional anxiety. I-CBT conceptualization examines how these responses inadvertently maintain reasoning errors rather than resolving underlying concerns.

Sarah's cleaning rituals temporarily reduce anxiety about contamination but reinforce the inference pattern by suggesting that elaborate precautions are necessary and that normal environmental conditions are dangerous.

Maintenance Mechanisms These are the cognitive and behavioral processes that keep obsessional patterns stable over time. Understanding maintenance helps identify what needs to change for recovery to occur.

Sarah's pattern is maintained by sensory distrust (dismissing evidence of cleanliness), possibility focus (treating remote risks as serious concerns), and intermittent reinforcement (occasional anxiety relief from cleaning confirms that rituals are "working").

Mapping Obsessional Narratives and Reasoning Stories

Every client with OCD develops characteristic "stories" that explain why their obsessional concerns are reasonable and necessary. These narratives feel completely logical from the inside but reveal systematic reasoning errors when examined objectively. Mapping these stories provides crucial insight into how obsessional thinking maintains itself.

The Structure of Obsessional Narratives

Obsessional stories typically follow a predictable structure that makes them feel compelling and difficult to dismiss:

Setup: Real-world situation with genuine uncertainty or responsibility
Escalation: Introduction of remote but theoretically possible negative outcomes
Amplification: Development of increasingly catastrophic consequences *Personalization:* Connection to vulnerable self-themes and identity concerns *Justification:* Explanation of why extraordinary precautions are reasonable

Marcus's door-checking narrative illustrates this structure clearly:

Setup: "I need to leave my apartment and want to make sure it's secure." *Escalation:* "What if the door isn't properly locked and someone breaks in?" *Amplification:* "If there's a break-in, valuable items could be stolen and my sense of security would be destroyed." *Personalization:* "If I failed to secure my home properly, what does that say about my competence as an independent adult?" *Justification:* "Given how much is at stake, spending extra time checking is just being responsible."

This narrative sounds reasonable on the surface, but I-CBT analysis reveals multiple reasoning errors: inverse inference (starting with break-in possibility), irrelevant association (treating apartment security like high-risk facility protection), and category errors (applying perfectionist standards to routine activities).

Identifying Story Elements

Effective narrative mapping requires identifying the specific elements that make each story feel compelling:

Core premises that the story treats as obviously true but actually represent reasoning errors *Emotional hooks* that connect practical concerns to vulnerable identity themes *Logical gaps* where the story jumps from possibility to probability without evidence *Maintenance loops* where story elements reinforce each other to create circular reasoning

Sarah's contamination narrative rests on several core premises that feel obviously true to her: "Dangerous germs could be anywhere," "I might not notice contamination," "My children depend on me for protection," and "Good mothers prevent all preventable risks." Each premise sounds reasonable but involves reasoning errors when examined closely.

The emotional hook connects practical hygiene concerns to profound questions about maternal adequacy. The logical gaps occur where Sarah jumps from "contamination is possible" to "contamination is likely" without considering base rates or evidence. The maintenance loop reinforces itself because cleaning rituals confirm that extraordinary precautions are necessary while providing temporary anxiety relief that validates the original concern.

Collaborative Story Analysis

Mapping obsessional narratives works best as a collaborative process where therapist and client work together to understand the logic of the obsessional story. This approach respects the client's intelligence while helping them see reasoning errors they haven't recognized.

The process typically begins with having the client tell their obsessional story in detail, including all the reasoning that makes their concerns feel important and necessary. The therapist listens carefully for reasoning patterns, vulnerable themes, and logical structure without immediately challenging the story's conclusions.

Next, the therapist helps the client identify the story's underlying premises and examine whether those premises are supported by evidence or represent reasoning assumptions. This analysis often reveals that stories which feel obviously true actually rest on foundations that can't be verified.

Finally, therapist and client work together to identify where the story diverges from evidence-based reasoning and how alternative stories might account for the same observations without requiring obsessional responses.

Identifying Vulnerable Self-Themes and Feared Possible Selves

Understanding vulnerable self-themes requires exploring the identity concerns that give obsessional thinking its emotional power. These themes represent areas where the client is particularly sensitive to doubt because they connect to fundamental aspects of how they see themselves and want to be seen by others.

Common Vulnerable Self-Themes

Research by O'Connor and Aardema identified several themes that frequently appear in obsessional thinking:

Competence and adequacy - Concerns about being capable, reliable, and effective in important roles and responsibilities *Moral character and goodness* - Questions about being an ethical, caring person who doesn't cause harm to others *Safety and protection* - Doubts about ability to keep oneself and loved ones safe from danger and harm *Cleanliness and acceptability* - Fears about being pure, clean, and socially acceptable to others *Precision and correctness* - Worries about doing things accurately and meeting appropriate standards

Most clients show primary and secondary themes, with obsessional episodes typically gravitating toward their most vulnerable areas regardless of how they begin.

Elena demonstrates a primary theme of maternal competence with secondary themes of family protection and moral character. Her contamination fears consistently lead to questions about whether she's an adequate mother who properly protects her children from harm.

Robert shows a primary theme of professional competence with secondary themes of precision and acceptability. His email checking behaviors reflect deep concerns about being seen as capable and reliable in his work relationships.

The Feared Possible Self

Vulnerable themes often center on what Aardema called the "feared possible self" - a version of identity that the person desperately wants to avoid becoming. This feared self represents the opposite of their ideal identity and serves as a powerful motivator for obsessional behaviors.

Sarah's feared possible self is "the neglectful mother who fails to protect her children and causes them to suffer needlessly." This feared identity drives her elaborate cleaning rituals because they feel like the only way to ensure she doesn't become that type of person.

Marcus's feared possible self is "the irresponsible adult who can't be trusted with basic life management." His checking behaviors serve to prove that he's careful and competent rather than careless and inadequate.

Understanding feared possible selves helps explain why obsessional behaviors feel so necessary and difficult to resist. The behaviors aren't just managing anxiety - they're actively constructing a preferred identity by avoiding a dreaded one.

Therapeutic Exploration of Themes

Exploring vulnerable themes requires sensitivity because these areas often involve the client's most important values and relationships. The goal isn't to challenge the importance of competence, morality, or safety, but to help clients recognize when reasonable concerns become obsessional preoccupations.

The exploration typically begins by identifying what matters most to the client in terms of their roles, relationships, and values. This discussion helps establish the themes that are genuinely important versus those that have become obsessionally exaggerated.

Next, the therapist helps the client examine how their obsessional thinking connects to these important themes. This analysis often reveals that obsessions represent distorted versions of healthy concerns rather than completely irrational fears.

Finally, the work focuses on distinguishing between reasonable attention to important themes versus obsessional preoccupation that actually interferes with living according to those values.

Treatment Planning Based on Assessment

I-CBT case conceptualization directly informs treatment planning by identifying specific reasoning errors, vulnerable themes, and intervention priorities for each individual client. This targeted approach improves treatment efficiency and outcomes compared to generic protocol application.

Module Selection and Sequencing

Different clients benefit from different combinations of I-CBT modules based on their reasoning profiles and vulnerable themes:

Clients with prominent *inverse inference* patterns benefit from early emphasis on evidence evaluation and reality sensing modules that help them distinguish observation from imagination.

Those showing strong *category errors* need focused work on contextual thinking and appropriate standard application.

Clients with *sensory distrust* require extensive reality sensing work before progressing to more advanced modules.

Those with elaborate *inference cascades* benefit from detailed chain analysis and interruption training.

Sarah's profile suggests she'll benefit from reality sensing modules (to address sensory distrust), evidence evaluation work (to correct irrelevant associations), and vulnerable theme exploration (to address maternal competence concerns). The sequencing should begin with psychoeducation about reasoning errors, progress through reality sensing training, and conclude with theme-based identity work.

Modification of Standard Protocols

While I-CBT follows a general 12-module framework, individual case conceptualizations often require protocol modifications to address specific reasoning patterns or life circumstances:

Pacing adjustments for clients who need more or less time to master specific concepts *Content modifications* to address cultural factors or unique vulnerable themes *Intensity variations* for clients with severe symptoms or limited therapy availability *Integration considerations* for those with significant comorbid conditions

Elena's conceptualization suggests she'll need extended work on modules addressing maternal themes, with possible integration of parenting stress management techniques. Her high insight and motivation suggest she can progress through psychoeducational modules relatively quickly.

Intervention Priority Setting

Case conceptualization helps establish intervention priorities when clients present with multiple obsessional themes or complex symptom patterns:

Primary themes that drive the most distress or functional impairment receive initial focus *Reasoning errors* that appear across multiple themes get prioritized over theme-specific concerns *Maintenance mechanisms* that keep the overall pattern stable become important intervention targets *Practical considerations* such as work demands or family responsibilities influence timing decisions

Marcus's conceptualization reveals that competence concerns drive both his checking behaviors and his work-related obsessions. Addressing the underlying competence theme will likely benefit multiple symptom areas more efficiently than targeting specific behaviors separately.

Template for I-CBT Case Formulation

The following template provides a structured framework for organizing I-CBT case conceptualizations:

Client Demographics and Presenting Concerns
- Basic identifying information
- Primary obsessional themes and symptoms
- Functional impairment and life impact
- Treatment goals and motivation level

Reasoning Error Profile
- Primary reasoning errors (inverse inference, category errors, etc.)
- Sensory trust versus imagination reliance patterns
- Evidence evaluation capabilities and limitations
- Inference chain development speed and complexity

Vulnerable Self-Theme Analysis
- Primary vulnerable themes and feared possible selves
- Connection between themes and obsessional content
- Historical development of theme sensitivity
- Current life circumstances affecting theme salience

Obsessional Narrative Structure
- Core premises underlying obsessional stories
- Emotional hooks connecting concerns to identity themes
- Logical gaps and reasoning jumps in narrative development
- Maintenance mechanisms sustaining narrative credibility

Trigger and Context Patterns
- Consistent environmental and internal triggers
- Situational factors that increase obsessional vulnerability

- Times, places, and circumstances associated with episodes
- Protective factors that reduce obsessional thinking

Treatment Planning Implications

- Recommended module sequence and emphasis areas
- Anticipated challenges and resistance points
- Integration needs with other therapeutic approaches
- Progress indicators and outcome measures

This template ensures that all relevant factors are considered while maintaining focus on the reasoning processes that I-CBT targets for intervention.

Three Complete Case Conceptualizations

Case Conceptualization 1: Jennifer - Contamination and Moral Responsibility

Demographics: Jennifer, 28, graduate student in social work, lives with roommate

Presenting Concerns: Elaborate hand-washing rituals (45 minutes multiple times daily), avoidance of public restrooms and public transportation, interference with academic and social functioning

Reasoning Error Profile: Primary inverse inference starting with disease transmission possibilities; strong irrelevant association connecting medical contamination information to everyday situations; moderate sensory distrust requiring extensive evidence to accept cleanliness

Vulnerable Self-Theme: Primary theme of moral responsibility and caring for others; feared possible self is "selfish person who spreads disease and harms innocent people"; secondary theme of professional competence in helping profession

Obsessional Narrative: "Dangerous pathogens exist everywhere and could be transmitted through casual contact. If I inadvertently spread disease to vulnerable people, I'm responsible for their suffering. As someone entering a helping profession, I have higher moral obligations to prevent harm. Normal hygiene standards aren't sufficient given the seriousness of potential consequences."

Treatment Planning: Begin with psychoeducation about reasoning errors, emphasize reality sensing and evidence evaluation modules, address moral responsibility themes in vulnerable self modules, integrate professional identity concerns

Case Conceptualization 2: David - Harm and Competence Concerns

Demographics: David, 35, software engineer, married with two young children

Presenting Concerns: Checking behaviors while driving (pulling over to verify no pedestrian impact), repeated verification of work product, excessive safety precautions with home appliances and tools

Reasoning Error Profile: Moderate inverse inference with strong possibility-probability confusion; prominent category errors applying perfectionist standards to routine activities; fast inference chain development creating rapid escalation to catastrophic concerns

Vulnerable Self-Theme: Primary theme of competence and reliability; feared possible self is "incompetent person who causes serious harm through carelessness"; secondary themes of family protection and professional adequacy

Obsessional Narrative: "Serious accidents can result from momentary inattention or minor mistakes. If I cause harm through inadequate checking or preparation, I'm responsible for preventable suffering. Competent people anticipate and prevent all reasonably possible negative outcomes. The consequences of being wrong are too serious to risk normal confidence levels."

Treatment Planning: Focus on possibility versus probability modules, extensive work on appropriate checking standards, address competence themes through professional and family role analysis, practice graduated risk acceptance

Case Conceptualization 3: Lisa - Social Acceptance and Perfectionism

Demographics: Lisa, 24, recent college graduate, working in marketing firm

Presenting Concerns: Excessive email and text message checking and rewriting, social media monitoring for negative responses, repeated analysis of social interactions for signs of disapproval

Reasoning Error Profile: Strong inverse inference starting with social rejection possibilities; prominent irrelevant association connecting normal social variation to personal inadequacy; slow inference chain development allowing detailed analysis of imagined social threats

Vulnerable Self-Theme: Primary theme of social acceptability and belongingness; feared possible self is "unlikeable person who is rejected and isolated"; secondary themes of professional competence and personal attractiveness

Obsessional Narrative: "Social relationships are fragile and require constant maintenance to prevent rejection. Minor social mistakes can have major consequences for relationship stability. If people think poorly of me, it reflects real inadequacies in my character or behavior. Successful people carefully monitor and manage their social image to prevent negative judgments."

Treatment Planning: Emphasize social evidence evaluation and reality sensing, address perfectionist standards in social contexts, work extensively on acceptance and belonging themes, practice social risk tolerance building

Practice Exercise: Formulation Development

The following case information provides an opportunity to practice I-CBT case conceptualization skills:

Background: Michael, 42, accountant, divorced, lives alone, has teenage daughter who visits weekends

Symptoms: Spends 2-3 hours each evening checking financial documents and calculations, repeatedly verifies that bills are paid correctly, excessive backup systems for important documents, anxiety about making mathematical errors that could have serious consequences

Assessment Information: High ICQ-EV score (28), Y-BOCS score of 24, significant work impairment, high insight into symptom unreasonableness, strong motivation for change

Client Statements: "I know I'm being excessive, but what if I make a mistake that costs me my job or damages my reputation? In my profession, accuracy is everything. One significant error could ruin my career and affect my ability to support my daughter."

Practice Tasks:

1. Identify Michael's primary reasoning errors
2. Determine his vulnerable self-themes and feared possible self
3. Map his obsessional narrative structure
4. Recommend treatment planning priorities
5. Predict potential challenges and resistance points

This exercise helps build skill in translating assessment information into actionable case conceptualizations that guide effective I-CBT treatment planning.

Integration with Ongoing Treatment

Case conceptualization in I-CBT is not a one-time assessment product but an evolving framework that develops throughout treatment. Initial conceptualizations provide starting points for intervention, but they require regular revision as new information emerges and the client develops insight into their reasoning patterns.

Ongoing conceptualization refinement serves several important functions:

Treatment modification based on emerging patterns or unexpected responses to intervention *Progress tracking* by documenting changes in reasoning errors and vulnerable theme sensitivity *Resistance analysis* when clients struggle with specific modules or concepts *Relapse prevention* by identifying persistent vulnerabilities that require ongoing attention

Sarah's case illustrates this evolution. Initial conceptualization focused on contamination fears and maternal competence themes. As treatment progressed, it became clear that her pattern also involved perfectionist standards and control concerns that weren't initially apparent. This recognition led to additional work on uncertainty tolerance and appropriate standard setting.

The collaborative nature of I-CBT conceptualization means that clients become active participants in understanding and refining their own reasoning patterns. This involvement enhances treatment engagement and helps clients develop skills for ongoing self-analysis beyond formal therapy.

Moving Toward Intervention

Comprehensive case conceptualization provides the foundation for effective I-CBT intervention by clarifying exactly what needs to change and how those changes can be achieved. Unlike symptom-focused approaches that target behavioral reduction, I-CBT conceptualization identifies specific reasoning errors and vulnerable themes that require attention.

This precision in targeting allows for more efficient treatment because interventions address underlying mechanisms rather than surface symptoms. When reasoning errors are corrected and vulnerable themes are appropriately addressed, symptom improvement typically follows naturally without requiring separate behavioral interventions.

The next chapter examines how to determine when I-CBT is the most appropriate treatment choice and how to navigate complex clinical situations where multiple treatment options might be considered.

Chapter 13: Differential Diagnosis and Treatment Selection

Dr. Patel reviews the intake information for three new clients scheduled for the week. Rebecca, 26, describes elaborate contamination rituals and cleaning behaviors that consume five hours daily. James, 31, experiences violent intrusive thoughts about harming family members and seeks constant reassurance about his character. Maya, 19, struggles with perfectionist checking behaviors but also reports severe depression, trauma history, and recent suicidal ideation.

Each case presents classic OCD symptoms, but they require completely different treatment approaches. Rebecca's clear reasoning errors and high insight make her an ideal candidate for I-CBT. James's violent obsessions might benefit from I-CBT but require careful assessment for overvalued ideation and risk factors. Maya's complex presentation needs stabilization and trauma work before any OCD-specific intervention can be safely attempted.

This scenario illustrates the critical importance of thoughtful treatment selection in OCD care. Not every person with obsessional symptoms benefits from the same approach, and I-CBT, despite its effectiveness, has specific indications and contraindications that must be carefully considered. Making appropriate treatment decisions requires understanding not just what I-CBT can accomplish, but when other approaches might be more suitable or necessary.

When to Choose I-CBT vs. Other Approaches

I-CBT represents one effective approach within a broader menu of evidence-based OCD treatments. Optimal treatment selection requires understanding the unique strengths and limitations of different approaches and matching them to individual client characteristics and circumstances.

I-CBT's Unique Strengths

I-CBT offers several advantages that make it particularly suitable for certain types of presentations:

Reasoning-focused intervention that addresses the cognitive mechanisms underlying obsessional thinking rather than just managing symptoms or reducing anxiety

High client acceptability because it doesn't require deliberate exposure to feared situations or prolonged anxiety tolerance

Educational approach that helps clients understand their condition and develop skills for long-term self-management

Preserved insight utilization that builds on the client's existing recognition that their fears are unreasonable rather than trying to overcome that insight

Identity integration that addresses the vulnerable self-themes and values that make obsessional concerns feel so compelling

Rebecca exemplifies an ideal I-CBT candidate. Her contamination fears rest on clear reasoning errors (treating household situations like medical environments), she maintains good insight into their unreasonableness, and she's motivated to understand why her thinking feels so compelling despite her intellectual recognition that her fears are excessive.

Traditional CBT/ERP Strengths

Exposure and Response Prevention (ERP) remains highly effective for many OCD presentations and offers distinct advantages in certain situations:

Behavioral focus that directly targets compulsive behaviors and avoidance patterns *Anxiety tolerance building* that helps clients function despite obsessional discomfort *Extensive research base*

supporting effectiveness across diverse OCD presentations *Structured protocols* that provide clear guidelines for implementation *Symptom reduction focus* that can provide rapid relief from severe behavioral symptoms

James might benefit more from traditional ERP approaches if his violent obsessions involve significant avoidance behaviors or if his reasoning patterns don't show clear errors. His concerns about character and morality might require behavioral testing through exposure rather than reasoning analysis.

Medication Considerations

Pharmacological interventions play important roles in comprehensive OCD treatment and sometimes represent the most appropriate initial intervention:

Severe symptom presentations that interfere with cognitive therapy participation *Significant comorbid depression* that affects motivation and concentration *Previous therapy failures* where medication might enhance psychological intervention effectiveness *Rapid symptom reduction needs* in crisis situations

Maya's complex presentation with severe depression and suicidal ideation likely requires pharmacological stabilization before any psychological intervention can be safely and effectively implemented.

Integration and Combination Approaches

Many clients benefit from combination treatments that utilize strengths of different approaches:

Sequential treatment where one approach addresses initial stabilization needs and another provides long-term improvement *Concurrent treatment* where medication supports psychological intervention effectiveness *Modular approaches* that combine elements from different therapeutic frameworks based on individual needs

Evidence-Based Selection Criteria

Research on treatment matching in OCD has identified several factors that predict differential response to various therapeutic approaches. These evidence-based criteria help guide clinical decision-making and improve treatment outcomes.

I-CBT Response Predictors

Studies by O'Connor, Aardema, and colleagues identified characteristics that predict positive response to I-CBT:

High inferential confusion scores (ICQ-EV > 20) indicate reasoning errors that I-CBT specifically targets

Preserved insight into symptom unreasonableness suggests intact reality testing that can be strengthened through reasoning work

Educational orientation where clients are curious about understanding their condition rather than just reducing symptoms

Motivation for reasoning change rather than pure symptom elimination

Specific obsessional themes including contamination, responsibility, and moral concerns that commonly involve reasoning errors

Moderate to severe symptoms that create motivation for change without overwhelming cognitive capacity

ERP Response Predictors

Traditional ERP approaches work best for clients with different characteristics:

Behavioral avoidance patterns that can be systematically addressed through graduated exposure

Anxiety tolerance deficits where building distress tolerance is the primary therapeutic need

Limited insight into symptom unreasonableness where behavioral change might precede cognitive change

Motivation for behavioral change regardless of underlying reasoning patterns

Specific presentations including symmetry obsessions and "just right" feelings that may have stronger biological components

Severe compulsive behaviors that require immediate behavioral intervention

Medication Response Predictors

Pharmacological interventions show better outcomes with certain presentations:

Severe symptom intensity that interferes with daily functioning and therapy participation

Significant comorbid depression that affects motivation and cognitive capacity

Family history of OCD suggesting stronger biological components

Early onset presentations that may involve more prominent neurobiological factors

Previous psychological treatment failures where medication might enhance therapy effectiveness

Research by Bloch and colleagues found that combination treatments often produce better outcomes than single-modality approaches, particularly for severe presentations with multiple comorbidities.

Contraindications and Limitations

While I-CBT shows effectiveness across diverse OCD presentations, certain factors suggest caution or alternative treatment selection. Understanding these limitations prevents inappropriate treatment recommendations and potential harm.

Absolute Contraindications

Active psychosis or severe reality testing problems that prevent distinguishing imagination from perception

Severe cognitive impairment that interferes with understanding abstract reasoning concepts

Active substance abuse that impairs cognitive function and therapy participation

Severe suicidal ideation requiring immediate crisis intervention and stabilization

Manic episodes where grandiosity and poor judgment affect treatment engagement

These conditions require stabilization before I-CBT can be safely and effectively implemented.

Relative Contraindications

Very low insight (poor recognition of symptom unreasonableness) that makes reasoning-focused work challenging

Severe overvalued ideation where clients truly believe their obsessional concerns are realistic

Significant intellectual limitations that affect comprehension of abstract concepts

Severe depression that impairs concentration and motivation

Recent trauma that requires processing before addressing obsessional symptoms

Cultural factors that conflict with I-CBT assumptions about reasoning and evidence

These factors don't absolutely preclude I-CBT but require careful consideration and possible treatment modifications.

Age-Related Considerations

I-CBT research has focused primarily on adult populations, and modifications are needed for different age groups:

Children and young adolescents may lack the abstract reasoning capacity necessary for traditional I-CBT concepts

Older adults with cognitive changes might struggle with complex reasoning analysis

Developmental factors affect both symptom presentation and treatment capacity

O'Connor and colleagues developed modified I-CBT protocols for adolescent populations, but pediatric applications require significant adaptation.

Comorbidity Considerations

Real-world OCD presentations frequently involve comorbid conditions that complicate treatment selection and implementation. Understanding how comorbidities interact with OCD symptoms helps guide appropriate treatment decisions.

Depression and OCD

Depression affects up to 60% of people with OCD and significantly impacts treatment planning:

Motivational effects where depression reduces engagement in challenging therapeutic work

Cognitive effects where depressed mood affects reasoning analysis and insight

Hopelessness that interferes with commitment to long-term treatment

Timing considerations regarding whether depression or OCD should receive initial treatment focus

Research suggests that moderate depression can be addressed concurrently with OCD treatment, but severe depression often requires initial stabilization before obsessional symptoms can be effectively targeted.

Maya's case illustrates these complexities. Her perfectionist checking behaviors involve clear reasoning errors suitable for I-CBT, but her severe depression and suicidal ideation require immediate attention. The treatment plan should address safety and depression stabilization before introducing reasoning-focused work.

Trauma and OCD

Trauma history appears in approximately 40% of OCD cases and creates specific treatment challenges:

Hypervigilance that makes reality sensing techniques more difficult

Trust issues that affect therapeutic relationship development

Trauma-related triggers that can activate both trauma responses and obsessional thinking

Complex symptom interactions where trauma and OCD symptoms reinforce each other

Post-traumatic stress often requires specific treatment before I-CBT can be effectively implemented. However, some trauma presentations benefit from I-CBT approaches that help distinguish realistic from exaggerated threat assessment.

Autism Spectrum Conditions and OCD

Autism spectrum conditions co-occur with OCD at higher than expected rates and create unique treatment considerations:

Social communication differences that affect therapy engagement and concept understanding

Sensory processing variations that complicate reality sensing work

Cognitive flexibility limitations that make reasoning change more challenging

Special interests that might overlap with obsessional themes

Executive function differences affecting treatment planning and homework completion

I-CBT can be effective for autistic individuals with OCD, but it requires significant modifications in communication style, concept presentation, and treatment pacing.

Managing Treatment-Resistant Cases

Some clients don't respond to initial I-CBT implementation despite appropriate selection criteria. Understanding potential causes of treatment resistance helps guide modifications and alternative approaches.

Common Sources of Resistance

Incomplete reasoning error identification where assessment missed crucial cognitive patterns

Unaddressed vulnerable themes that weren't recognized during initial evaluation

Hidden overvalued ideation where clients truly believe some obsessional concerns are realistic

Motivation ambivalence where clients want symptom relief but resist reasoning change

Life circumstances that maintain stress levels and trigger obsessional episodes

Therapeutic relationship factors affecting engagement and collaboration

Resistance Assessment and Modification

When I-CBT progress stalls, systematic assessment can identify modification needs:

Reasoning pattern re-evaluation to identify missed cognitive factors

Vulnerable theme exploration to uncover identity concerns not initially apparent

Motivation assessment to understand ambivalence about change

Environmental factor analysis to identify maintaining circumstances

Therapeutic process review to address relationship or technique factors

Robert's case illustrates resistance modification. Initial I-CBT focused on his email checking behaviors and perfectionist standards. When progress stalled, reassessment revealed unaddressed competence concerns related to childhood criticism and current work stress. Adding vulnerable theme work and stress management improved treatment response.

When to Consider Alternative Approaches

Sometimes I-CBT resistance indicates that different treatment approaches might be more appropriate:

Persistent reasoning error patterns despite adequate I-CBT implementation might suggest neurobiological factors requiring medication

Overwhelming anxiety that prevents reasoning analysis might benefit from ERP approaches that build distress tolerance

Complex trauma affecting reasoning capacity might require trauma-focused treatment before addressing OCD

Severe behavioral symptoms might need immediate behavioral intervention before reasoning work

Family factors maintaining obsessional patterns might require family therapy approaches

Decision Algorithm for Treatment Selection

The following decision framework helps organize treatment selection considerations:

Step 1: Safety and Stability Assessment

- Assess for immediate safety concerns (suicidality, severe depression)
- Evaluate cognitive capacity and reality testing
- Identify crisis factors requiring immediate intervention

Step 2: Symptom Pattern Analysis

- Administer ICQ-EV and other assessment tools
- Identify primary reasoning errors and vulnerable themes
- Assess insight levels and motivation for change

Step 3: Comorbidity Evaluation

- Screen for depression, anxiety, trauma, and other conditions
- Determine whether comorbidities require concurrent or sequential treatment
- Assess how comorbidities might affect I-CBT implementation

Step 4: Treatment Matching

- High ICQ-EV scores + good insight + reasoning-focused motivation = I-CBT indicated
- Significant behavioral avoidance + anxiety tolerance deficits = consider ERP
- Severe depression + cognitive impairment = consider medication first
- Complex presentation = consider combination or sequential approaches

Step 5: Implementation Planning

- Modify protocols for individual factors (age, culture, comorbidities)
- Plan for resistance assessment and treatment modification
- Establish progress monitoring and decision points for approach changes

Ethical Considerations in Treatment Choice

Treatment selection decisions involve important ethical considerations that affect client welfare and professional responsibility.

Informed Consent Requirements

Clients deserve clear information about:

- Evidence base for different treatment options
- Expected benefits and potential risks of each approach
- Treatment duration and intensity requirements
- Alternatives available if initial treatment doesn't work

This information should be presented in understandable language without overwhelming clients with excessive detail or creating paralysis around decision-making.

Competence and Training Considerations

Therapists should only provide treatments for which they have adequate training and competence:

- Formal I-CBT training through approved programs
- Supervised experience with inference-based approaches
- Ongoing consultation for complex cases
- Recognition of competence limitations and appropriate referral

Cultural Sensitivity and Appropriateness

Treatment selection should consider:

- Cultural beliefs about mental health and treatment
- Language and communication preferences
- Family and community factors affecting treatment participation
- Religious or spiritual beliefs that might interact with reasoning-focused work

Economic and Practical Factors

Ethical treatment selection considers:

- Insurance coverage and financial accessibility
- Geographic availability of trained therapists
- Time and scheduling constraints affecting treatment participation
- Transportation and childcare factors

These practical considerations shouldn't override clinical appropriateness but need integration into treatment planning to ensure realistic and sustainable treatment implementation.

Integration with Stepped Care Models

I-CBT fits well within stepped care approaches that match treatment intensity to individual needs and progress through increasingly intensive interventions as needed.

Step 1: Education and Self-Help

- Bibliotherapy and online resources about reasoning patterns
- Self-assessment tools for identifying reasoning errors
- Basic reality sensing and evidence evaluation techniques

Step 2: Brief Intervention

- Short-term I-CBT modules focusing on specific reasoning errors
- Group treatment formats for common presentations
- Consultation models for less severe symptoms

Step 3: Standard I-CBT Treatment

- Full 18-24 session individual treatment protocol
- Comprehensive reasoning analysis and vulnerable theme work
- Standard module progression with individual modifications

Step 4: Intensive Intervention

- Intensive outpatient programs incorporating I-CBT
- Combination treatments with medication and other approaches
- Specialized programs for complex or treatment-resistant cases

This stepped approach ensures that clients receive appropriate treatment intensity while preserving more intensive resources for those who need them most.

Future Directions in Treatment Selection

Ongoing research continues to refine treatment selection criteria and develop new approaches for improving matching between clients and interventions.

Emerging Assessment Tools

- Neuroimaging predictors of treatment response
- Genetic markers affecting medication response
- Cognitive testing for reasoning capacity assessment

- Cultural adaptation measures

Treatment Innovations

- Technology-enhanced I-CBT delivery
- Cultural adaptations for diverse populations
- Integration with mindfulness and acceptance approaches
- Precision medicine approaches using multiple predictors

Implementation Research

- Training models for widespread I-CBT dissemination
- Healthcare system integration strategies
- Cost-effectiveness comparisons across approaches
- Long-term outcome tracking and maintenance

These developments will continue to improve the precision and effectiveness of treatment selection while making evidence-based interventions more accessible to diverse populations.

Building Clinical Judgment

Effective treatment selection ultimately depends on skilled clinical judgment that integrates evidence-based criteria with individual client factors and circumstances. This judgment develops through training, experience, and ongoing consultation with colleagues.

Key elements of sound clinical judgment include:

- Thorough assessment using appropriate tools
- Understanding of evidence base and treatment mechanisms
- Recognition of one's own competence limitations
- Flexibility to modify approaches based on client response
- Commitment to ongoing learning and skill development

The goal isn't to develop rigid decision rules but to build sophisticated clinical reasoning that serves each client's unique needs and circumstances while adhering to evidence-based principles and ethical guidelines.

Treatment selection represents just the beginning of the therapeutic process. Once appropriate treatment decisions are made, the real work begins: implementing effective interventions that help people recover from the reasoning errors that create obsessional suffering.

Chapter 14: Treatment Structure and the 12-Module Protocol

When Maria first sits down for her initial I-CBT session, she brings a thick folder of previous therapy notes, medication trials, and self-help worksheets from three years of treatment attempts. "I've tried everything," she says, exhaustion evident in her voice. "CBT, medications, exposure therapy, mindfulness - nothing seems to stick. The obsessions always come back."

Dr. Thompson nods with understanding, then opens a simple notebook to a clean page. "What we're going to do differently," she explains, "is follow a specific roadmap that targets exactly how your mind creates obsessional thinking. Instead of managing symptoms or building tolerance for anxiety, we're going to teach your brain to recognize when it's using imagination instead of evidence."

This conversation illustrates a fundamental shift that occurs when clients begin I-CBT treatment. Instead of facing another generic therapeutic approach, they encounter a structured, systematic protocol specifically designed to correct the reasoning errors that create obsessional suffering. The 12-module framework provides both therapist and client with a clear roadmap for recovery that targets precise cognitive mechanisms rather than attempting broad symptom management.

Understanding this treatment structure is crucial for effective I-CBT implementation. The modules build progressively, each one preparing the client for more advanced concepts while addressing specific aspects of obsessional reasoning. This systematic approach ensures that no critical elements are missed while allowing for individualized pacing and modification based on each client's unique presentation and needs.

Overview of 18-24 Session Treatment Course

I-CBT typically requires 18-24 individual sessions spread over 4-6 months, though this timeline can be adjusted based on symptom severity, individual learning pace, and life circumstances. This duration reflects the time needed for clients to master new reasoning skills and apply them consistently across different situations and obsessional themes.

The treatment course is deliberately structured to allow progressive skill building without overwhelming clients with too much information too quickly. Research by O'Connor and colleagues found that shorter treatment courses often result in incomplete learning, while longer courses may reduce motivation and delay the confidence-building that comes from independent application of skills.

Phase 1: Foundation Building (Sessions 1-6) The initial phase focuses on assessment, psychoeducation, and introducing basic I-CBT concepts. Clients learn to recognize their own reasoning patterns and understand how obsessional thinking differs from normal problem-solving. This phase emphasizes collaboration and hope-building as clients begin to see their symptoms as correctable reasoning errors rather than mysterious mental illness.

Phase 2: Core Skill Development (Sessions 7-15) The middle phase introduces the primary I-CBT interventions including reality sensing, evidence evaluation, and inference chain interruption. Clients practice these skills extensively with therapist guidance before attempting independent application. This phase typically produces the most dramatic symptom improvements as clients learn to recognize and interrupt obsessional reasoning in real-time.

Phase 3: Integration and Relapse Prevention (Sessions 16-24) The final phase focuses on consolidating gains, addressing vulnerable themes, and preparing for long-term maintenance of improvements.

Clients learn to handle setbacks, recognize early warning signs of reasoning errors, and maintain their gains without ongoing therapeutic support.

The session frequency typically begins with weekly meetings during the foundation and skill development phases, then transitions to biweekly and eventually monthly sessions during the integration phase. This graduated reduction in contact helps clients build confidence in their independent application of I-CBT principles.

Elena's treatment course illustrates typical progression. Her contamination obsessions responded well to reality sensing and evidence evaluation work in sessions 8-12, with significant symptom reduction occurring over just four weeks. However, she needed additional sessions (16-22) to address underlying maternal competence themes that became apparent once her surface symptoms improved.

The 12-Module Progression Framework

The I-CBT protocol consists of 12 distinct modules that can be completed in 18-24 sessions depending on individual pacing needs. Some modules require only one session, while others may span 2-3 sessions for complex presentations or slower learning pace.

Modules 1-3: Understanding the Foundation These modules establish the conceptual foundation by helping clients understand how obsessional thinking develops and operates. Clients learn to map their own inference chains and recognize the difference between evidence-based and imagination-based reasoning.

Module 1: The Obsessional Sequence introduces the basic trigger-to-compulsion progression and helps clients identify their personal patterns.

Module 2: The Logic Behind OCD teaches the five major reasoning errors that drive obsessional thinking and helps clients recognize these patterns in their own experience.

Module 3: Constructing the Obsessional Story helps clients understand how their mind creates compelling narratives that justify obsessional behaviors despite lack of supporting evidence.

Modules 4-6: Challenging Core Assumptions These modules target the fundamental assumptions that make obsessional thinking feel reasonable and necessary. Clients learn to distinguish between legitimate concerns and imagination-based fears.

Module 4: The Vulnerable Self explores the identity themes that give obsessional thinking its emotional power and helps clients recognize when reasonable self-concern becomes obsessional preoccupation.

Module 5: OCD is 100% Imaginary demonstrates that obsessional concerns lack direct evidence and exist entirely in the realm of theoretical possibility rather than observable reality.

Module 6: Doubt and Possibility teaches clients to distinguish between realistic uncertainty that can be resolved through investigation and obsessional doubt that persists despite evidence.

Modules 7-9: Building Alternative Responses These modules provide practical tools for responding differently to triggers and obsessional thoughts. Clients learn active techniques for staying grounded in reality rather than getting pulled into imagination-based scenarios.

Module 7: The OCD Bubble helps clients recognize when they've entered the alternate reality of obsessional thinking and provides techniques for returning to evidence-based awareness.

Module 8: Reality Sensing teaches specific skills for gathering and trusting sensory evidence rather than relying on imagination or theoretical concerns.

Module 9: Creating Different Stories helps clients develop alternative, evidence-based narratives that account for their observations without requiring obsessional responses.

Modules 10-12: Integration and Maintenance These final modules consolidate learning and prepare clients for long-term maintenance of their gains. The focus shifts from learning new skills to preventing relapse and handling challenging situations independently.

Module 10: Tricks of the OCD Con Artist helps clients recognize the subtle ways obsessional thinking tries to regain control and provides techniques for resisting these manipulations.

Module 11: Developing the Real Self focuses on strengthening authentic identity and values that aren't dependent on obsessional behaviors or perfect certainty.

Module 12: Relapse Prevention teaches clients to recognize early warning signs, handle setbacks appropriately, and maintain their gains over time.

Session-by-Session Roadmap

While individual pacing varies, the following roadmap provides a typical progression through I-CBT treatment:

Sessions 1-2: Assessment and Introduction Complete comprehensive assessment including ICQ-EV, Y-BOCS, and reasoning pattern analysis. Introduce basic I-CBT concepts and begin Module 1 if time permits. Establish therapeutic rapport and collaborative treatment goals.

Sessions 3-4: Obsessional Sequence Mapping Complete Module 1 with detailed mapping of client's specific inference chains. Begin Module 2 with introduction to reasoning error categories. Assign homework to track obsessional episodes between sessions.

Sessions 5-6: Reasoning Error Recognition Complete Module 2 with extensive practice identifying reasoning errors in client's own thinking patterns. Begin Module 3 with exploration of obsessional story structure. Introduce concept of cross-over from evidence to imagination.

Sessions 7-8: Story Construction and Vulnerable Themes Complete Module 3 with detailed analysis of client's obsessional narratives. Begin Module 4 with exploration of vulnerable self-themes and feared possible selves. This transition often produces significant insight and emotional processing.

Sessions 9-10: Imagination vs. Reality Complete Module 4 with thorough examination of identity concerns underlying obsessional thinking. Begin Module 5 with demonstration that obsessional concerns lack direct evidence. This module often produces dramatic shifts in perspective.

Sessions 11-12: Doubt and Possibility Work Complete Module 5 with extensive evidence evaluation exercises. Begin and often complete Module 6 focusing on the difference between realistic and obsessional doubt. Clients typically show significant behavioral changes during this period.

Sessions 13-14: Reality Sensing Skills Begin Module 7 with OCD bubble concept and techniques for recognizing when thinking has shifted to imagination. Begin Module 8 with extensive reality sensing practice. These skills require considerable practice to master.

Sessions 15-16: Alternative Story Development Complete Module 8 with advanced reality sensing applications. Begin Module 9 with practice creating evidence-based alternative stories for typical triggering situations. Homework emphasizes real-world application.

Sessions 17-18: Advanced Integration Complete Module 9 and begin Module 10 focusing on OCD's manipulation tactics. Clients practice recognizing subtle forms of obsessional thinking that might not be immediately obvious. Problem-solve challenging situations that have emerged during treatment.

Sessions 19-21: Identity and Self Development Complete Module 10 and work extensively on Module 11 addressing authentic self-development and values-based living. This work often reveals deeper themes that require additional processing time.

Sessions 22-24: Relapse Prevention and Termination Complete Module 11 and focus primarily on Module 12 relapse prevention strategies. Plan for termination and discuss booster session scheduling. Review progress and celebrate achievements while preparing for independent maintenance.

Pacing and Adaptation Guidelines

Effective I-CBT implementation requires flexibility in pacing while maintaining the logical progression of concepts. Some clients master modules quickly and can progress rapidly, while others need extended time to understand and apply specific concepts.

Factors Affecting Pacing

Baseline insight levels significantly affect how quickly clients can progress through psychoeducational modules. Those with high insight often move rapidly through Modules 1-3, while those with limited insight may need extended time to recognize their reasoning patterns.

Cognitive capacity and processing speed influence how much information can be covered in each session. Some clients benefit from slower presentation with extensive repetition and practice.

Emotional intensity and anxiety levels can interfere with learning new concepts. Highly anxious clients may need more time to process information and practice new skills.

Life circumstances and stressors affect both session attendance and homework completion. Clients facing major life changes may need extended treatment timelines or modified expectations.

Comorbid conditions such as depression or attention problems can slow learning and require adapted presentation methods.

Adaptation Strategies

When clients struggle with specific modules, several adaptation approaches can help:

Extended time allows more practice with challenging concepts before progressing to advanced material.

Simplified presentation breaks complex concepts into smaller, more manageable pieces.

Alternative examples may resonate better with clients who don't connect with standard case illustrations.

Modified homework assignments can accommodate different learning styles and life circumstances.

Increased frequency of sessions may help clients who struggle with retention between weekly meetings.

Marcus illustrates successful adaptation. His initial difficulty understanding the difference between evidence and imagination (Module 5) led to spending three sessions on this concept instead of the typical one. This extended time was crucial because his entire treatment success depended on mastering this fundamental distinction.

Warning Signs of Pacing Problems

Several indicators suggest that pacing adjustments may be needed:

Repeated confusion about concepts that should have been mastered in previous sessions *Inability to complete homework assignments* despite apparent motivation *Increasing anxiety or resistance* as treatment progresses *Lack of behavioral change* despite reported understanding of concepts *Frequent requests to review previous material* instead of progressing forward

When these patterns appear, it's often better to slow down and ensure solid foundation skills rather than pushing forward with advanced concepts that won't be effectively utilized.

Individual vs. Group Delivery Options

I-CBT can be delivered effectively in both individual and group formats, each offering distinct advantages and considerations for different client populations and practice settings.

Individual Treatment Advantages

Personalized pacing allows adaptation to each client's learning style and processing speed *Detailed assessment* can identify subtle reasoning patterns that might be missed in group settings *Flexible scheduling* accommodates work and family obligations more easily *Privacy protection* for clients uncomfortable sharing personal obsessional content *Intensive focus* on individual vulnerable themes and specific reasoning errors

Individual treatment typically provides the most thorough and personalized intervention, particularly for complex presentations or clients with significant comorbidities.

Group Treatment Advantages

Cost effectiveness makes treatment accessible to more people *Peer support* reduces isolation and provides modeling of recovery *Shared learning* allows clients to recognize reasoning errors more easily in others before identifying them in themselves *Efficiency* for therapists serving larger caseloads *Reduced stigma* through recognition that others struggle with similar reasoning patterns

Research by Aardema and colleagues found that group I-CBT can be as effective as individual treatment for appropriately selected clients, particularly those with good insight and similar reasoning error patterns.

Hybrid Approaches

Many clinicians combine individual and group elements:

Assessment and initial sessions conducted individually, followed by group treatment for core modules *Group treatment* for educational modules (1-6) followed by individual work on vulnerable themes (7-

12) *Primary group treatment* with individual booster sessions as needed

Group Selection Criteria

Effective group treatment requires careful client selection:

Similar insight levels prevent some group members from feeling overwhelmed or frustrated *Compatible reasoning error patterns* allow shared focus on relevant concepts *Adequate verbal communication skills* for group participation *Willingness to share personal examples* and engage in group discussions *Stable mental state* without active crisis issues that would dominate group attention

Visual Treatment Timeline

Creating visual timelines helps both therapists and clients understand the treatment progression and maintain motivation during challenging periods. These timelines can be customized for individual presentations while maintaining the basic I-CBT structure.

Standard Timeline Visual Elements

Assessment phase (Sessions 1-2) shown as foundation building with emphasis on understanding current patterns *Education phase* (Sessions 3-8) illustrated as skill acquisition with focus on learning new concepts *Application phase* (Sessions 9-16) depicted as active practice with real-world implementation *Integration phase* (Sessions 17-24) shown as independence building with reduced therapist dependence

Customized Timeline Features

Individual timelines should highlight: *Personal milestones* such as first successful inference chain interruption or reality sensing application *Anticipated challenges* based on individual reasoning patterns and vulnerable themes *Celebration points* where significant progress typically occurs *Support reminders* during periods when motivation commonly drops

Sarah's timeline showed anticipated rapid progress during reality sensing modules (Sessions 11-14) followed by expected challenges during vulnerable theme work (Sessions 17-20) as maternal competence concerns became focus of treatment.

Progress Tracking Integration

Visual timelines work best when integrated with ongoing progress tracking: *ICQ-EV scores* plotted over time to show reasoning improvement *Y-BOCS scores* tracking symptom reduction *Functional improvement markers* such as return to avoided activities *Confidence ratings* in applying I-CBT skills independently

Common Modifications and Adaptations

Real-world I-CBT implementation often requires modifications to accommodate individual needs, cultural factors, and practical constraints. Understanding common adaptation patterns helps therapists maintain treatment effectiveness while adjusting for unique circumstances.

Cultural and Linguistic Adaptations

Language modifications for non-native English speakers may require simplified terminology and extensive use of examples *Cultural reasoning patterns* that differ from Western logic models need acknowledgment and integration *Family involvement* expectations vary across cultures and may require modified approaches *Religious or spiritual beliefs* about uncertainty, control, and responsibility require sensitive integration

Age-Related Modifications

Adolescent adaptations require more concrete examples and shorter attention spans for complex concepts *Older adult modifications* may need accommodation for cognitive changes and different life priorities *Developmental considerations* affect both concept understanding and homework completion capacity

Comorbidity Adaptations

Depression modifications may require slower pacing and motivation enhancement strategies *Autism spectrum adaptations* often need more concrete examples and modified social communication approaches *ADHD accommodations* might include shorter sessions and modified homework assignments

Practical Constraint Adaptations

Insurance limitations may require compressed treatment timelines or group delivery *Geographic barriers* might necessitate telehealth delivery or intensive formats *Work schedule conflicts* could require evening or weekend sessions *Childcare constraints* might require flexible scheduling or family involvement

Jennifer's treatment illustrates successful adaptation. Her autism spectrum diagnosis required concrete examples, written summaries of each session, and extended time for processing new concepts. Her treatment took 28 sessions instead of the typical 20, but achieved excellent outcomes through patient, adapted implementation.

Intensive Treatment Formats

Some clients benefit from intensive delivery formats that compress the timeline:

Daily sessions over 2-3 weeks for clients who can take time off work *Weekend workshops* covering multiple modules in extended sessions *Retreat formats* combining intensive treatment with peer support *Hybrid intensive approaches* with daily sessions followed by weekly maintenance

Research suggests that intensive formats can be as effective as standard weekly treatment for motivated clients without significant comorbidities.

Treatment Structure Success Factors

Several factors consistently predict successful I-CBT implementation across different settings and client populations:

Clear Communication of Structure Clients who understand the treatment progression and rationale show better engagement and outcomes. Taking time to explain the module framework and expected timeline pays dividends in motivation and compliance.

Flexible Adherence to Progression While the module sequence shouldn't be dramatically altered, successful therapists adapt pacing and emphasis based on individual client needs and responses.

Homework Integration The treatment structure works best when clients actively practice concepts between sessions through structured homework assignments that build progressively.

Progress Monitoring Regular assessment using ICQ-EV and other measures helps identify when clients are ready to progress versus when additional time is needed on specific concepts.

Therapist Training and Support Effective implementation requires adequate training in the I-CBT model and ongoing consultation for challenging cases.

Understanding treatment structure provides the foundation for effective I-CBT delivery. The 12-module framework offers a proven roadmap for helping clients develop the reasoning skills necessary for lasting recovery from obsessional thinking patterns.

The next chapter begins detailed exploration of the first three modules, showing exactly how to implement the foundational concepts that make all subsequent I-CBT work possible.

Chapter 15: Modules 1-3 - Understanding the Obsessional Sequence

Rachel sits in session 3, staring at the whiteboard where Dr. Kim has drawn a simple flowchart: Trigger → Doubt → Consequence → Anxiety → Compulsion. "That's it?" Rachel asks, sounding almost disappointed. "That's what's been controlling my life for eight years?" Dr. Kim nods. "It seems simple when you see it laid out like this, but your mind makes it feel incredibly complex and urgent. Learning to see this pattern clearly is the first step to interrupting it."

This moment captures the power of the initial I-CBT modules. What feels like mysterious, overwhelming mental chaos to the client becomes a clear, predictable sequence that can be mapped, understood, and eventually interrupted. Modules 1-3 establish the foundation for all subsequent I-CBT work by helping clients recognize that their obsessions follow specific patterns rather than representing random psychological attacks.

These foundational modules serve multiple therapeutic functions beyond simple education. They begin shifting the client's relationship with their symptoms from helpless victim to informed observer. They establish hope by demonstrating that obsessional thinking operates by understandable rules. Most importantly, they provide the conceptual framework necessary for clients to benefit from the more advanced interventions introduced in later modules.

Module 1: Introducing the Obsessional Sequence

The first module focuses on helping clients recognize that their obsessional experiences follow a predictable sequence that can be mapped and analyzed. This may seem obvious to therapists familiar with CBT models, but many clients experience obsessions as chaotic, unpredictable events that seem to come from nowhere and spiral out of control.

Core Learning Objectives for Module 1

Clients should be able to identify the five stages of obsessional sequences in their own experience, recognize that obsessions follow patterns rather than occurring randomly, and begin to see themselves as observers of their thinking rather than passive victims of their symptoms.

Typical Session Structure

The session typically begins with reviewing any homework from previous sessions, then introduces the obsessional sequence concept through psychoeducation and personal examples. The middle portion involves collaborative mapping of the client's specific sequences, and the session concludes with homework assignment and preview of upcoming work.

Introducing the Sequence Concept

Most clients benefit from starting with a general explanation before examining their personal patterns:

"Most people think OCD is about anxiety or fear, but it's actually about a specific type of thinking that follows the same pattern over and over. Today we're going to map that pattern so you can see exactly how your mind creates obsessional episodes."

The therapist then introduces the five-stage sequence using neutral, non-threatening examples before moving to the client's specific experiences. This approach reduces defensiveness and helps clients see the pattern more clearly.

The Five-Stage Progression

Stage 1: Trigger - Something real and observable that starts the sequence. This could be external (seeing something, hearing a sound, encountering a situation) or internal (a thought, feeling, or bodily sensation). The key point is that triggers are always based on something that actually occurs.

Stage 2: Obsessional Doubt - The initial "what if" thought that crosses over from reality to imagination. This doubt typically sounds reasonable on the surface but involves treating remote possibilities as serious concerns.

Stage 3: Imagined Consequence - The mind immediately jumps to potential negative outcomes if the doubt proves true. These consequences often escalate quickly from minor problems to catastrophic scenarios.

Stage 4: Anxiety Response - The body responds to the imagined consequences as if they were real threats, generating the physical and emotional discomfort that makes the doubts feel so compelling.

Stage 5: Compulsive Response - Behaviors (mental or physical) designed to reduce anxiety or prevent the imagined consequences from occurring.

Collaborative Sequence Mapping

The heart of Module 1 involves working with clients to map their specific obsessional sequences. This process requires patience and careful questioning to help clients recognize patterns they may never have consciously identified.

Marcus provides a clear example of this collaborative mapping process:

Therapist: "Can you think of a recent obsessional episode that we could map together?"

Marcus: "Yesterday I was leaving my apartment and suddenly got really anxious about whether I locked the door."

Therapist: "Let's start with the trigger. What exactly happened right before you started worrying about the lock?"

Marcus: "I was walking down the hallway toward the elevator."

Therapist: "So the trigger was the physical act of walking away from your door. What was the first doubt that came to mind?"

Marcus: "I thought, 'What if I didn't actually lock it? What if I just thought I locked it but didn't really do it?'"

Therapist: "And what did your mind tell you would happen if the door wasn't locked?"

Marcus: "Someone could break in, steal my stuff, or worse. I could come home to find everything destroyed."

The mapping continues through anxiety response (heart racing, sweating, feeling of dread) and compulsive response (returning to check the lock multiple times). This detailed analysis helps Marcus see that his "random" anxiety actually follows a specific, predictable pattern.

Common Challenges in Module 1

Many clients initially struggle to distinguish between triggers and doubts, often reporting that obsessional thoughts appear "out of nowhere." Patient exploration usually reveals specific triggers that the client hadn't consciously recognized.

Some clients resist the idea that their concerns follow predictable patterns, feeling that this minimizes the real importance of their worries. The therapist should validate that the concerns feel important while helping the client see that understanding patterns is the first step toward addressing them effectively.

Other clients become overly focused on the content of their obsessions rather than the process. The therapist should gently redirect attention from whether specific concerns are valid to how the thinking pattern operates.

Module 2: The Logic Behind OCD (Five Reasoning Categories)

While Module 1 helps clients map the sequence of obsessional episodes, Module 2 examines the specific reasoning errors that drive this sequence. Understanding these "tricks" that OCD uses helps clients recognize when their thinking has shifted from evidence-based to imagination-based.

The Five Major Reasoning Categories

O'Connor and Aardema identified five primary reasoning errors that appear consistently across different obsessional presentations:

Category 1: Inverse Inference - Starting with feared outcomes and working backward to current concerns rather than starting with current evidence and reasoning forward to logical conclusions.

Category 2: Irrelevant Associations - Connecting accurate information to situations where that information doesn't apply or isn't relevant.

Category 3: Category Errors - Applying standards, information, or principles from one context to inappropriate situations.

Category 4: Over-Reliance on Possibility - Treating theoretical possibilities as practical concerns that require immediate attention.

Category 5: Distrust of Senses - Dismissing clear sensory evidence in favor of imagined alternatives or theoretical concerns.

Teaching Through Examples

Each reasoning category is best understood through concrete examples that clients can relate to their own experience:

Inverse Inference Example: "Instead of looking at the door and seeing that it's locked, your mind starts with the possibility of break-in and works backward: 'If someone breaks in, the door would have to be unlocked. Since break-ins are possible, maybe my door isn't really locked.'"

Irrelevant Association Example: "You read that hospital-acquired infections are a serious problem and then start worrying about germs in your kitchen. The medical information is accurate, but it applies to hospital settings with sick patients, not your home environment."

The therapist should use examples from the client's own experience whenever possible, helping them recognize these reasoning patterns in their specific obsessions.

Interactive Reasoning Analysis

Module 2 works best when clients actively participate in identifying reasoning errors rather than passively receiving information. The therapist might present scenarios and ask clients to identify which reasoning errors are operating:

"Sarah reads that E. coli outbreaks sometimes occur in restaurants and then starts worrying about the chicken she cooked at home last night. What reasoning errors might be happening here?"

This interactive approach helps clients develop skill in recognizing reasoning errors in real-time, which becomes crucial for later intervention modules.

Resistance and Validation Issues

Some clients resist the idea that their reasoning contains errors, feeling that this invalidates their concerns or suggests they're "stupid." The therapist should emphasize that these reasoning errors are:

- Universal human tendencies that everyone experiences occasionally
- Specific to obsessional themes rather than reflecting general intelligence
- Understandable responses to uncertainty and anxiety
- Correctable patterns rather than permanent deficits

The goal is helping clients recognize reasoning errors without feeling criticized or defensive about their thinking patterns.

Module 3: Constructing the Obsessional Story

Module 3 builds on the sequence mapping and reasoning error identification to help clients understand how their minds construct elaborate narratives that make obsessional behaviors feel reasonable and necessary. These stories feel completely logical from the inside but reveal systematic reasoning errors when examined objectively.

Understanding Obsessional Narratives

Every client develops characteristic "stories" that explain why their obsessional concerns are important and why their compulsive responses are justified. These narratives typically include:

- Explanation of why the concern is realistic and important
- Description of potential consequences if precautions aren't taken
- Justification for why extraordinary measures are reasonable
- Connection to personal values and identity themes

Elena's contamination story illustrates this pattern:

"Dangerous germs exist everywhere and could harm my children. Normal cleaning might miss invisible contamination that could make them seriously ill. As a responsible mother, I have to do everything possible to protect them. If I don't clean thoroughly and something happens, I'll never forgive myself."

This narrative sounds reasonable on the surface, but I-CBT analysis reveals multiple reasoning errors: irrelevant association (applying medical contamination information to home settings), over-reliance on possibility (treating remote risks as serious concerns), and category errors (applying hospital-level hygiene standards to domestic situations).

Collaborative Story Analysis

The therapist and client work together to identify the elements of the client's obsessional stories:

Story premises - What assumptions does the story treat as obviously true? *Logical connections* - How does the story link initial concerns to final conclusions? *Emotional hooks* - What values or identity themes make the story feel compelling? *Evidence gaps* - Where does the story jump from possibility to probability without supporting evidence?

This analysis helps clients recognize that their obsessional stories, while internally consistent, rest on foundations of reasoning errors rather than solid evidence.

Alternative Story Development

Once clients can see the structure of their obsessional stories, Module 3 introduces the concept of alternative narratives based on evidence rather than imagination:

Elena's alternative story: "Normal household environments contain typical germs that healthy immune systems handle routinely. Standard hygiene practices provide adequate protection for family health. Good parenting includes reasonable precautions without excessive anxiety that interferes with family life."

The alternative story accounts for the same observations (germs exist, children need protection) but draws different conclusions based on evidence rather than theoretical possibilities.

Detailed Session Guides with Scripts

Effective Module 1-3 implementation requires specific therapeutic language and techniques that help clients grasp these foundational concepts without feeling overwhelmed or criticized.

Module 1 Session Script Elements

Opening: "Today we're going to map exactly how your obsessional episodes develop. This will help you see that what feels chaotic and unpredictable actually follows specific patterns."

Transition to mapping: "Let's pick a recent episode and trace it step by step. Try to choose something that happened in the last few days so the details are still clear."

Sequence identification: "What exactly triggered this episode? Was it something you saw, heard, felt, or thought? Let's be very specific about what actually happened."

Doubt exploration: "What was the first 'what if' thought that came to mind? This is usually where your thinking shifted from observing reality to imagining possibilities."

Consequence development: "Once that doubt appeared, what did your mind tell you might happen? How did the consequences build from that initial worry?"

Response analysis: "What did you do to handle the anxiety or prevent the imagined consequences? How did that response affect your thoughts and feelings?"

Module 2 Script Elements

Concept introduction: "Now that you can see your obsessional sequence, let's examine the specific thinking tricks your mind uses to make imaginary concerns feel real and urgent."

Reasoning error explanation: "These aren't signs that you're irrational or unintelligent. They're specific reasoning patterns that everyone uses occasionally, but OCD makes them stronger and more frequent in certain situations."

Personal application: "Looking at the episode we mapped yesterday, which of these reasoning errors do you notice in your own thinking?"

Validation and normalization: "It makes perfect sense that your mind would use these reasoning shortcuts when you're anxious or uncertain. The goal isn't to eliminate all reasoning errors, but to recognize when they're leading you into obsessional territory."

Client Handouts and Worksheets

Effective implementation of Modules 1-3 requires structured handouts and worksheets that reinforce session learning and provide frameworks for between-session practice.

Module 1 Worksheet: Obsessional Sequence Mapping

Trigger (What actually happened?):

_____

Obsessional Doubt (First "what if" thought):

_____

Imagined Consequences (What your mind said might happen):

_____

Anxiety Response (Physical and emotional reactions):

_____

Compulsive Response (What you did to handle the anxiety):

_____

Cross-over Point (Where did your thinking shift from evidence to imagination?):

_____

Module 2 Handout: Reasoning Error Quick Reference

Inverse Inference: Starting with feared outcome instead of current evidence *Irrelevant Association:* Applying information to inappropriate situations *Category Error:* Using wrong standards for the situation *Over-Reliance on Possibility:* Treating "could happen" as "will happen" *Sensory Distrust:* Ignoring clear evidence in favor of imagination

Module 3 Worksheet: Story Analysis

My Obsessional Story:

What are the main premises of my story?

What values or identity themes does it connect to?

Where does it jump from possibility to probability?

What reasoning errors does it include?

Alternative Evidence-Based Story:

What do the facts actually show?

What would normal concern look like in this situation?

How would someone without OCD think about this?

What story fits the evidence without requiring compulsions?

Role-Play Scenarios for Practice

Therapist training in Modules 1-3 benefits from extensive role-play practice with common client presentations and challenging scenarios.

Scenario 1: Contamination Obsessions *Client role:* "I don't understand how washing my hands for safety is an obsession. Germs are real, and my children could get sick." *Therapist practice:* Validate concern about family health while exploring reasoning patterns and helping client see difference between reasonable hygiene and obsessional cleaning.

Scenario 2: Harm Obsessions *Client role:* "But what if I really am dangerous? What if these thoughts mean I'm capable of hurting someone?" *Therapist practice:* Distinguish between having thoughts and acting on them while mapping the reasoning sequence that transforms normal protective instincts into obsessional doubt.

Scenario 3: Responsibility Obsessions *Client role:* "I know checking seems excessive, but what if something happens because I wasn't careful enough?" *Therapist practice:* Explore appropriate vs. excessive responsibility while helping client recognize reasoning errors that make normal checking feel insufficient.

Troubleshooting Common Challenges

Several challenges commonly arise during Modules 1-3 that require specific therapeutic responses:

Challenge: Client can't identify specific triggers *Response:* Use recent, detailed examples and explore the moments immediately before obsessional thoughts began. Many triggers are subtle and require careful examination to identify.

Challenge: Client insists concerns are realistic *Response:* Acknowledge that concerns often contain elements of realistic worry while focusing on the reasoning process rather than content validity. "The question isn't whether contamination is possible, but how your mind moves from possibility to compelling urgency."

Challenge: Client becomes overwhelmed by analysis *Response:* Slow down and focus on one clear example rather than trying to analyze multiple episodes. Emphasize that understanding patterns takes time and practice.

Challenge: Client resists homework assignments *Response:* Explore resistance collaboratively and modify assignments to match client's capacity and comfort level. Start with simple observation tasks before moving to detailed analysis.

Challenge: Client wants to skip to "solutions" *Response:* Explain that these foundational modules are necessary for later interventions to be effective. "We need to understand exactly how the problem works before we can fix it effectively."

Building the Foundation for Advanced Work

Modules 1-3 establish the conceptual foundation that makes all subsequent I-CBT interventions possible. Clients who master these foundational concepts typically progress smoothly through later modules, while those who struggle with the basics often have difficulty with advanced techniques.

The key indicators of successful Module 1-3 completion include:

- Clear recognition of personal obsessional sequence patterns
- Ability to identify reasoning errors in their own thinking
- Understanding that obsessions involve imagination rather than evidence
- Beginning shift from passive victim to active observer of their thinking
- Motivation to learn tools for interrupting obsessional reasoning

These foundational modules transform the client's relationship with their symptoms from mysterious, overwhelming forces to understandable patterns that can be analyzed and modified. This shift in perspective creates the hope and motivation necessary for the challenging work ahead in Modules 4-6, where clients begin directly challenging their obsessional thinking patterns.

Chapter 16: Modules 4-6 - Vulnerable Self and Imagination

When David completes Module 3, he feels a mix of excitement and apprehension. "I can see my checking pattern now," he tells Dr. Rivera. "Trigger, doubt, catastrophe, anxiety, compulsion. It's like clockwork. But here's what I don't understand - if I know it's just a pattern, why does it still feel so important? Why does the thought of not checking feel dangerous, even when I intellectually know it's unnecessary?"

Dr. Rivera smiles. "That's exactly the right question, and it leads us to the heart of what makes obsessional thinking so compelling. Your checking isn't really about door locks or stove knobs. It's about something much deeper - your sense of yourself as a competent, responsible person. When OCD attacks that core identity, the behaviors feel necessary regardless of logic."

This conversation illustrates the transition from understanding obsessional mechanics (Modules 1-3) to addressing the deeper identity concerns that fuel emotional intensity (Modules 4-6). These modules represent the most psychologically challenging portion of I-CBT treatment because they explore the vulnerable self-themes that make obsessional thinking feel so compelling and difficult to resist.

Modules 4-6 accomplish several critical therapeutic goals: they help clients understand why their obsessions feel so emotionally important, demonstrate that obsessional concerns exist entirely in imagination rather than evidence, and teach clients to distinguish between realistic uncertainty and obsessional doubt. This work often produces dramatic symptom improvements as clients realize their behaviors are protecting imaginary rather than real concerns.

Module 4: The Vulnerable Self-Theme and Feared Possible Self

Module 4 represents a significant shift in I-CBT focus from analyzing thinking patterns to understanding the identity concerns that make those patterns feel emotionally compelling. Most clients quickly grasp that their obsessions follow specific sequences, but they struggle to understand why breaking those sequences feels so threatening to their sense of self.

Understanding Vulnerable Self-Themes

Vulnerable self-themes represent core identity areas where people are particularly sensitive to doubt because these areas connect to their most important values, relationships, and sense of personal adequacy. Research by Aardema and O'Connor identified several themes that commonly appear in obsessional thinking:

Competence and adequacy - Concerns about being capable, reliable, and effective in important roles *Moral character and goodness* - Questions about being ethical, caring, and trustworthy *Safety and protection* - Doubts about ability to keep oneself and loved ones safe *Cleanliness and acceptability* - Fears about being pure, appropriate, and socially acceptable *Precision and correctness* - Worries about doing things accurately and meeting standards

These themes aren't arbitrary - they typically reflect the client's genuine values and priorities. The problem occurs when reasonable concern in these areas becomes obsessional preoccupation that interferes with effective functioning.

The Feared Possible Self

Within each vulnerable theme lies what Aardema called the "feared possible self" - a version of identity that the person desperately wants to avoid becoming. This feared self represents the antithesis of their ideal identity and serves as a powerful motivator for obsessional behaviors.

Sarah's feared possible self is "the negligent mother who fails to protect her children and causes them unnecessary suffering." This feared identity drives her elaborate cleaning rituals because they feel like the only way to ensure she doesn't become that type of person.

Marcus's feared possible self is "the irresponsible adult who can't handle basic life management and creates problems through carelessness." His checking behaviors serve to prove that he's careful and competent rather than careless and inadequate.

Understanding feared possible selves helps explain why obsessional behaviors feel so necessary and difficult to resist. The behaviors aren't just managing anxiety - they're actively constructing a preferred identity by avoiding a dreaded one.

Therapeutic Exploration Techniques

Module 4 requires sensitive exploration because vulnerable themes often involve the client's most important values and relationships. The goal isn't to challenge the importance of competence, morality, or safety, but to help clients recognize when reasonable concerns become obsessional preoccupations.

Values clarification helps distinguish between healthy attention to important themes versus obsessional preoccupation: "What does being a good parent actually involve? How would you recognize good parenting in someone else?"

Behavioral analysis examines whether obsessional behaviors actually support or interfere with living according to important values: "Do your cleaning rituals help you be a better mother, or do they take time away from activities that would benefit your children?"

Alternative identity exploration helps clients recognize that their core identity doesn't depend on obsessional behaviors: "What would you think about a friend who was a caring mother but didn't spend three hours cleaning each day?"

Common Themes and Presentations

Different vulnerable themes typically connect to specific types of obsessional presentations:

Competence themes often appear in checking behaviors, perfectionist concerns, and work-related obsessions. Clients fear being seen as careless, unreliable, or inadequate.

Moral character themes frequently involve harm obsessions, religious scrupulosity, and relationship concerns. Clients worry about being bad, selfish, or harmful people.

Safety themes commonly manifest in protection rituals, avoidance behaviors, and contamination fears. Clients feel responsible for preventing all possible harm to themselves or others.

Acceptability themes often involve social obsessions, appearance concerns, and contamination fears. Clients worry about being disgusting, inappropriate, or rejected by others.

Resistance and Defensiveness

Module 4 often generates resistance because exploring vulnerable themes can feel threatening or embarrassing. Several therapeutic strategies help navigate this resistance:

Normalization emphasizes that everyone has areas of vulnerability and sensitivity *Validation* acknowledges that the themes represent genuine, important values *Collaboration* involves clients as experts on their own experience and values *Gentle pacing* allows time to process emotional content without overwhelming clients

Elena initially resisted exploring her maternal competence themes: "I don't want to talk about being a bad mother. That's not what this is about." The therapist responded: "You're absolutely right that you're not a bad mother. That's exactly the point - your cleaning rituals are trying to solve a problem that doesn't actually exist."

Module 5: OCD is 100% Imaginary (Lacks Direct Evidence)

Module 5 represents one of the most powerful and often transformative components of I-CBT treatment. It systematically demonstrates that obsessional concerns, despite feeling urgent and important, exist entirely in the realm of imagination and theoretical possibility rather than observable evidence.

The Imagination vs. Evidence Distinction

The core insight of Module 5 is helping clients recognize that obsessional thinking operates entirely through imagination rather than evidence. This doesn't mean the concerns are "made up" or unimportant to the client, but that they're based on theoretical possibilities rather than observable facts.

Evidence-based thinking starts with observable information and draws reasonable conclusions from available data. If you see that the door is locked, feel the deadbolt in position, and hear the mechanism click, you conclude the door is secure.

Imagination-based thinking starts with theoretical possibilities and treats them as if they require serious consideration regardless of contradictory evidence. Even when you can see, feel, and hear that the door is locked, imagination insists that "maybe it's not really secure."

Systematic Evidence Analysis

Module 5 involves systematic examination of the client's obsessional concerns to demonstrate their imaginary nature:

Direct evidence assessment - "What observable evidence supports your contamination concern? What can you actually see, touch, smell, or measure that indicates danger?"

Indirect evidence evaluation - "What signs or symptoms would appear if your concern were valid? Are any of those signs actually present?"

Contradictory evidence recognition - "What evidence contradicts your obsessional concern? How does your mind dismiss or explain away this contradictory information?"

Marcus provides a clear example of this analysis:

Obsessional concern: "The door might not be properly locked." *Direct evidence:* "I can see the deadbolt extended, feel it in the locked position, and hear it engage when I turn the key." *Contradictory evidence:* "I've checked this lock hundreds of times and it's never actually been unlocked when I thought it might be." *Imagination component:* "But what if this time is different? What if the mechanism is faulty? What if I didn't turn the key far enough?"

This analysis reveals that Marcus's concern exists entirely in imagination - there's no observable evidence supporting it, and abundant evidence contradicting it.

The Possibility Trap

Module 5 addresses what researchers call the "possibility trap" - the tendency to treat theoretical possibilities as practical concerns requiring action. This trap is particularly powerful because possibilities can rarely be completely eliminated, making them seem legitimate regardless of probability.

Realistic possibility assessment involves considering likelihood, evidence, and context: "While contamination is theoretically possible anywhere, what does the evidence suggest about this specific situation?"

Obsessional possibility inflation treats remote possibilities as serious concerns: "Because contamination is possible, I must treat every situation as if it's contaminated until proven otherwise."

The key therapeutic insight is helping clients recognize that infinite possibilities exist in any situation, but normal functioning requires responding to probabilities based on evidence rather than possibilities based on imagination.

Demonstration Exercises

Module 5 often includes experiential exercises that demonstrate the distinction between evidence and imagination:

Reality testing involves carefully examining evidence for and against obsessional concerns in real-time situations.

Possibility generation exercises help clients recognize how many theoretical concerns could be invented for any situation, demonstrating the arbitrary nature of obsessional focus.

Evidence comparison directly contrasts the amount and quality of evidence supporting versus contradicting obsessional concerns.

Sarah's contamination fears illustrate effective demonstration:

Exercise: Examine the kitchen counter that triggered her last cleaning episode *Evidence for contamination:* No visible contamination, no unusual odors, no family illness despite normal use *Evidence against contamination:* Clean appearance, normal household environment, effective previous cleaning *Possibility inflation:* "But invisible germs could be present that I can't detect" *Reality check:* "What evidence would actually support treating this as a contaminated surface?"

Module 6: Doubt and Possibility (Irrelevance Without Evidence)

Module 6 builds on the imagination versus evidence distinction to help clients understand the fundamental difference between realistic uncertainty that can be resolved through investigation and obsessional doubt that persists regardless of evidence.

Understanding Obsessional Doubt

Obsessional doubt differs qualitatively from normal uncertainty in several key ways:

Evidence resistance - Normal doubt decreases when relevant evidence is gathered; obsessional doubt persists or increases despite contradictory evidence

Regenerative quality - Normal doubt gets resolved and stays resolved; obsessional doubt keeps returning even after being addressed

Disproportionate urgency - Normal doubt matches the importance of the situation; obsessional doubt creates crisis-level urgency about minor concerns

Infinite expansion - Normal doubt has natural boundaries; obsessional doubt can generate endless new angles and concerns

The Certainty Trap

Many clients believe their obsessional behaviors are attempts to achieve reasonable certainty about important matters. Module 6 reveals that obsessional doubt doesn't actually seek certainty - it seeks an impossible guarantee that can never be provided.

Reasonable certainty accepts that perfect knowledge isn't always possible or necessary and makes decisions based on adequate information.

Obsessional certainty demands require guarantees that no situation can provide and refuse to accept any level of uncertainty as tolerable.

Robert's email checking illustrates this distinction:

Reasonable certainty: "I've proofread this email twice and it communicates my message clearly. That's adequate for workplace correspondence."

Obsessional certainty: "I need to be absolutely certain there are no errors, unclear phrases, or possible misinterpretations that could damage my professional reputation."

The first approach accepts normal uncertainty about how others will interpret communication. The second demands an impossible guarantee that all possible misunderstandings be prevented.

Possibility Without Evidence

Module 6 teaches clients to recognize when their concerns are based on possibilities that lack supporting evidence. This distinction is crucial because possibilities can be endlessly generated for any situation, making them seem legitimate simply because they can be imagined.

Evidence-supported possibilities have observable factors that increase their likelihood: "The weather forecast shows storm conditions, so power outages are possible."

Evidence-free possibilities exist only because they can be theoretically imagined: "Power outages are always possible, so I should prepare for one every day."

The therapeutic goal is helping clients distinguish between possibilities worth considering (those with supporting evidence) and possibilities that represent obsessional thinking (those without evidence but with emotional charge).

Doubt Assessment Techniques

Module 6 provides specific techniques for evaluating whether doubt represents realistic uncertainty or obsessional thinking:

The Evidence Test: "What observable information supports this concern? What contradicts it?"

The Resolution Test: "When you've addressed this concern before, did it stay resolved or keep returning?"

The Proportionality Test: "Does the intensity of your concern match the actual importance of this situation?"

The Possibility Test: "Are you responding to evidence or just to the fact that something is theoretically possible?"

Elena's maternal competence doubts illustrate effective doubt assessment:

Concern: "Maybe I'm not being careful enough about my children's safety." *Evidence test:* "What specific evidence suggests inadequate care? What evidence contradicts this concern?" *Resolution test:* "When you've reassured yourself about safety before, did the worry stay gone or return?" *Proportionality test:* "Does your level of worry match actual risk factors in your children's environment?" *Possibility test:* "Are you responding to actual safety indicators or to the theoretical possibility of harm?"

Therapeutic Techniques for Each Module

Successful implementation of Modules 4-6 requires specific therapeutic techniques adapted to the unique challenges of each module's content.

Module 4 Techniques

Values clarification helps distinguish healthy concern from obsessional preoccupation by exploring what the client actually wants to achieve in vulnerable theme areas.

Behavioral cost-benefit analysis examines whether obsessional behaviors help or hinder living according to important values.

Identity flexibility work helps clients recognize that their core worth doesn't depend on perfect performance in vulnerable areas.

Compassionate self-observation teaches clients to observe their vulnerable themes with kindness rather than harsh self-criticism.

Module 5 Techniques

Evidence inventory systematically catalogs observable information for and against obsessional concerns.

Reality testing exercises involve careful examination of actual conditions rather than imagined possibilities.

Possibility deflation helps clients recognize the arbitrary nature of focusing on remote possibilities while ignoring probable realities.

Imagination labeling teaches clients to recognize when thinking has shifted from evidence analysis to possibility speculation.

Module 6 Techniques

Doubt classification helps clients distinguish realistic uncertainty from obsessional doubt through systematic evaluation.

Certainty reality checking examines whether the level of certainty being demanded is realistic or reasonable for the situation.

Evidence requirement clarification helps establish appropriate standards for decision-making that don't require impossible guarantees.

Uncertainty normalization teaches acceptance of normal ambiguity as part of healthy functioning.

Case Examples of Successful Implementation

Case Example 1: Jennifer's Contamination Recovery

Jennifer's vulnerable theme centered on being a responsible, caring person who doesn't harm others through negligence. Her feared possible self was "selfish person who spreads disease and hurts innocent people."

Module 4 work revealed that her cleaning rituals actually interfered with caring behaviors by consuming time and energy she could spend helping others.

Module 5 work demonstrated that her contamination concerns lacked any observable evidence - no illness, no visible contamination, no medical reason for concern.

Module 6 work helped her recognize that her doubts about cleanliness persisted regardless of evidence and demanded impossible guarantees about disease prevention.

Outcome: Jennifer reduced hand-washing from 45 minutes to normal duration within six weeks, recognizing that her behaviors protected imaginary rather than real concerns.

Case Example 2: David's Checking Resolution

David's vulnerable theme involved competence and adequacy as an independent adult. His feared possible self was "irresponsible person who creates problems through carelessness."

Module 4 work revealed that excessive checking actually demonstrated anxiety rather than competence and interfered with effective life management.

Module 5 work showed that his security concerns lacked evidence - no break-ins, functional locks, safe neighborhood conditions.

Module 6 work helped him distinguish between reasonable security measures and obsessional doubt that demanded impossible certainty.

Outcome: David eliminated repetitive checking within eight weeks, recognizing that competent adults trust evidence rather than demanding perfect certainty.

Homework Assignments and Review

Modules 4-6 require structured homework assignments that help clients apply session concepts to real-world situations between therapeutic contacts.

Module 4 Homework

Values versus behaviors inventory - List important values in vulnerable theme areas and evaluate whether current behaviors support or interfere with those values.

Feared self exploration - Write detailed description of feared possible self and examine whether obsessional behaviors actually prevent or create that outcome.

Alternative identity modeling - Observe others who embody healthy versions of important values without obsessional behaviors.

Module 5 Homework

Evidence logging - Track observable evidence for and against obsessional concerns over one week.

Possibility generation - Practice identifying multiple theoretical possibilities for neutral situations to demonstrate arbitrary nature of obsessional focus.

Reality checking - Test specific obsessional predictions against actual outcomes.

Module 6 Homework

Doubt classification - Categorize daily doubts as realistic uncertainty versus obsessional doubt using assessment criteria.

Certainty demand examination - Identify situations where you're demanding impossible guarantees versus accepting normal uncertainty.

Evidence requirement clarification - Establish reasonable standards for decision-making in vulnerable areas.

Managing Resistance and Engagement

Modules 4-6 often generate significant resistance because they challenge core beliefs and identity concerns that clients may be reluctant to examine. Several strategies help manage this resistance while maintaining therapeutic progress.

Resistance to Vulnerable Theme Work

Some clients resist exploring vulnerable themes because it feels too personal or threatening. Effective responses include:

Normalizing vulnerability - Everyone has areas of sensitivity; exploring them is part of understanding how OCD operates *Emphasizing choice* - Clients control how much personal information to share *Connecting to symptoms* - Vulnerable themes explain why obsessions feel so compelling and difficult to resist *Validating values* - The themes represent important, legitimate concerns that deserve healthy attention

Resistance to Imagination Analysis

Some clients resist accepting that their concerns are imagination-based because it feels invalidating or dismissive. Helpful approaches include:

Clarifying terminology - "Imagination-based" doesn't mean unimportant or made up *Emphasizing mechanism* - Understanding how obsessions work helps address them effectively *Validating distress* - Imagination-based concerns can cause real suffering *Focusing on freedom* - Recognizing imagination allows choice about how to respond

Engagement Enhancement Strategies

Collaborative exploration - Work with clients as partners in understanding their experience *Personal relevance* - Connect concepts to specific examples from client's life *Gradual progression* - Build understanding slowly rather than rushing through concepts *Regular check-ins* - Monitor comprehension and emotional comfort throughout process

Building Toward Reality Sensing

Modules 4-6 prepare clients for the reality sensing and intervention work of Modules 7-9 by establishing crucial foundations:

- Understanding that obsessions protect imaginary rather than real concerns

- Recognition that vulnerable themes can be addressed through healthy rather than obsessional means

- Distinction between evidence-based and imagination-based thinking

- Skills for evaluating doubt and uncertainty appropriately

Clients who master Modules 4-6 typically show significant motivation for learning practical intervention techniques because they understand why such techniques are necessary and how they can restore healthy functioning in important life areas.

The transformation often evident after Module 6 completion represents one of I-CBT's most powerful outcomes: clients shift from feeling helplessly controlled by mysterious mental forces to understanding that they can choose evidence-based responses to life's normal uncertainties.

Chapter 17: Modules 7-9 - Reality Sensing and Alternative Narratives

After completing Module 6, Lisa sits quietly for several minutes, processing what she's learned. "So you're telling me," she finally says, "that all this anxiety about my social media posts isn't based on any actual evidence of rejection? That I'm basically living in an imaginary world where normal social interactions become threats?" Dr. Santos nods. "Exactly. And now that you can see you're operating in imagination rather than reality, we can teach you specific skills for staying grounded in what's actually happening rather than what your mind invents might be happening."

This conversation marks the transition from understanding obsessional mechanisms to learning practical intervention skills. Modules 7-9 represent the action phase of I-CBT treatment, where clients acquire specific techniques for interrupting obsessional reasoning and staying connected to evidence-based reality.

These modules often produce the most dramatic behavioral changes in I-CBT treatment because they provide concrete tools for managing obsessional episodes as they occur. Instead of being passive victims of obsessional thinking, clients become active agents who can recognize when their minds have shifted into imagination mode and redirect attention back to observable evidence.

Module 7: The OCD Bubble (Alternate Reality)

Module 7 introduces one of I-CBT's most powerful concepts: the idea that obsessional thinking creates an alternate reality - the "OCD bubble" - that feels completely real but operates by different rules than evidence-based reality.

Understanding the OCD Bubble

The OCD bubble represents a psychological space where theoretical possibilities feel more compelling than observable facts, where remote risks seem more important than actual conditions, and where imagination carries more weight than sensory evidence. When someone enters this bubble, normal reasoning processes become distorted in predictable ways.

Inside the OCD bubble:

- Possibilities feel like probabilities
- Theoretical concerns seem more important than actual evidence
- Remote risks appear to justify immediate action
- Sensory information gets dismissed in favor of imagined alternatives
- Normal uncertainty becomes intolerable crisis

Outside the OCD bubble:

- Evidence guides decision-making
- Probabilities matter more than possibilities
- Current information takes precedence over theoretical concerns
- Sensory data provides reliable guidance
- Normal uncertainty is acceptable and manageable

Recognizing Bubble Entry

Learning to recognize when thinking has shifted into the OCD bubble is crucial for effective intervention. Several warning signs typically indicate bubble entry:

Emotional intensity that seems disproportionate to the actual situation *Urgency* about theoretical concerns that lack supporting evidence *Sensory dismissal* where clear evidence gets ignored in favor of imagined possibilities *Catastrophic thinking* that jumps quickly from minor concerns to major disasters *Compulsive urgency* where specific actions feel absolutely necessary

Marcus learns to recognize his bubble entry signals: "It's like a switch flips in my brain. Suddenly the door lock that looked perfectly secure a minute ago seems unreliable. I can see it's locked, but that doesn't matter anymore - what matters is all the ways it might not be working properly."

Bubble vs. Reality Comparison

Module 7 works best when clients can directly compare their bubble thinking with reality-based thinking about the same situation:

Bubble perspective: "The stove might be on even though it looks off. The control knob might not be working properly. A gas leak could start a fire that destroys the building."

Reality perspective: "The stove appears off, the control knob is in the off position, and there's no smell of gas. The likelihood of malfunction is extremely low, and normal people don't repeatedly check appliances."

This comparison helps clients recognize how dramatically their perception changes when they enter the bubble, even though the actual situation remains identical.

Therapeutic Bubble Work

Effective bubble work requires helping clients recognize their specific bubble patterns without making them feel criticized for having distorted thinking:

Pattern identification - "What are the first signs that you've entered the bubble? What changes in your thinking or feeling?"

Reality anchoring - "When you notice bubble thinking, what evidence can anchor you back in observable reality?"

Bubble interruption - "What techniques help you step back and evaluate whether you're responding to evidence or imagination?"

The goal isn't to prevent all bubble entry (which may be impossible) but to develop quick recognition and effective exit strategies.

Module 8: Reality Sensing Techniques

Module 8 provides the practical heart of I-CBT intervention by teaching specific techniques for staying connected to evidence-based reality rather than getting pulled into imagination-based concerns.

Core Reality Sensing Principles

Reality sensing operates on several key principles that distinguish it from anxiety management or thought-stopping techniques:

Evidence primacy - Observable information takes precedence over theoretical possibilities *Sensory trust* - Direct perception provides more reliable information than imagination *Present focus* - Current conditions matter more than past fears or future worries *Contextual awareness* - Normal standards apply to normal situations

These principles help clients make appropriate decisions based on actual conditions rather than imagined scenarios.

The 5-4-3-2-1 Grounding Technique

One of the most practical reality sensing tools involves systematic engagement with all five senses to anchor attention in current, observable reality:

5 things you can see - Specific, detailed visual observations *4 things you can touch* - Textures, temperatures, pressures you can feel *3 things you can hear* - Sounds present in your environment *2 things you can smell* - Any scents or odors currently detectable *1 thing you can taste* - Flavors present in your mouth

This technique works because it systematically shifts attention from imagination-based concerns to evidence-based observations.

Elena practices 5-4-3-2-1 during kitchen anxiety:

See: Clean dishes, clear water, organized counter, normal lighting, soap bubbles dissipating *Touch:* Smooth dish surfaces, warm water, soft towel texture, solid counter *Hear:* Water running, dishes clinking, normal household sounds, her own breathing *Smell:* Fresh dish soap, clean water, absence of unusual odors *Taste:* Normal mouth taste, no unusual flavors

This inventory reveals that all sensory evidence supports cleanliness and normal conditions, contradicting her contamination concerns.

Advanced Reality Sensing Applications

As clients master basic reality sensing, they can learn more sophisticated applications:

Probability assessment - Using evidence to evaluate realistic likelihood rather than theoretical possibility *Contextual evaluation* - Considering normal standards for the specific situation rather than applying inappropriate criteria *Evidence comparison* - Weighing supporting versus contradicting information objectively *Temporal grounding* - Focusing on current conditions rather than past concerns or future fears

Integration with Daily Activities

Reality sensing works best when integrated into normal daily routines rather than used only during crisis moments:

Routine reality checks during regular activities like cooking, driving, or working *Preventive sensing* when approaching known trigger situations *Maintenance sensing* to stay connected to evidence throughout the day *Recovery sensing* after obsessional episodes to return to evidence-based awareness

Robert integrates reality sensing into his email routine: "Before I start checking for the third time, I use reality sensing to evaluate what I actually observe about the email's clarity and completeness. Usually this shows me that further checking isn't needed."

Module 9: Creating Different Stories

Module 9 builds on reality sensing skills to help clients develop alternative narratives based on evidence rather than imagination. Instead of trying to suppress obsessional stories, clients learn to construct better stories that account for the same observations without requiring compulsive responses.

Alternative Story Principles

Effective alternative stories share several characteristics:

Evidence-based - They start with observable information rather than theoretical possibilities *Proportional* - The response matches the actual situation rather than imagined scenarios *Contextually appropriate* - They apply normal standards to normal situations *Functionally adaptive* - They support effective life functioning rather than interference

Story Construction Process

Creating alternative stories involves systematic analysis of the situation from an evidence-based perspective:

Step 1: Observe current evidence - What can you actually see, hear, feel, smell, or measure?

Step 2: Consider normal explanations - What would most people conclude from this evidence?

Step 3: Apply appropriate standards - What level of certainty or action does this situation realistically require?

Step 4: Check proportionality - Does your response match the actual importance and likelihood of concerns?

Step 5: Test functionality - Does this story support effective living or create unnecessary interference?

Practical Story Development

Sarah's contamination alternative story illustrates effective construction:

Obsessional story: "Kitchen surfaces might harbor dangerous pathogens that could sicken my family. I must clean extensively to prevent illness and protect my children."

Alternative story: "Normal kitchen environments contain typical bacteria that healthy immune systems handle routinely. Standard cleaning practices provide adequate protection. Excessive cleaning takes time away from family activities without providing meaningful additional safety."

The alternative story accounts for the same concerns (germs exist, family health matters) but draws different conclusions based on evidence rather than imagination.

Story Testing and Refinement

Alternative stories work best when tested against real-world outcomes:

Prediction making - Use the alternative story to predict what will happen if you follow evidence-based responses *Outcome tracking* - Monitor results to see whether alternative stories lead to better or worse outcomes than obsessional stories *Story adjustment* - Refine alternative narratives based on actual experience rather than theoretical concerns

Lisa tests her social media alternative story: "Instead of analyzing every comment for hidden rejection, I'll assume normal social interaction unless clear evidence suggests otherwise." Tracking outcomes over several weeks shows improved relationships and reduced anxiety without negative social consequences.

Core Intervention Strategies

Modules 7-9 introduce several intervention strategies that clients can use independently to manage obsessional episodes as they occur.

Bubble Recognition and Exit

Early warning systems help clients recognize bubble entry before obsessional thinking becomes overwhelming *Reality anchors* provide specific techniques for reconnecting with evidence-based thinking *Exit strategies* offer structured approaches for leaving the bubble when recognition occurs

Evidence Evaluation Protocols

Systematic evidence review provides frameworks for objectively assessing obsessional concerns *Contradictory evidence emphasis* helps clients notice information that challenges obsessional narratives *Evidence versus imagination sorting* teaches clients to distinguish between observable facts and theoretical possibilities

Alternative Response Development

Evidence-based action planning helps clients determine appropriate responses based on actual rather than imagined conditions *Proportional response matching* ensures that actions fit the realistic importance of situations *Functional outcome optimization* focuses on responses that support effective living rather than anxiety reduction

Experiential Exercises for Sessions

Modules 7-9 work best when clients practice techniques during sessions rather than just discussing them theoretically.

Bubble Recognition Exercise

Have the client describe a recent obsessional episode in detail, then help them identify:

- The moment when thinking shifted from evidence to imagination
- How their perception of the situation changed after bubble entry
- What evidence was ignored or dismissed during bubble thinking
- How the situation looks different from outside the bubble

Reality Sensing Practice

Guide the client through 5-4-3-2-1 exercises using trigger situations:

- Start with neutral situations to build skill
- Progress to mildly triggering situations
- Practice during actual obsessional episodes if possible
- Emphasize the contrast between sensory evidence and imagined concerns

Story Construction Workshop

Work collaboratively to develop alternative stories for the client's typical obsessional themes:

- Start with the client's current obsessional narrative
- Identify evidence-based observations within that narrative
- Construct alternative explanations based solely on evidence
- Test alternative stories against real-world outcomes

Building Client Skills Progressively

Effective implementation of Modules 7-9 requires careful attention to skill progression, ensuring that clients master basic concepts before attempting advanced applications.

Phase 1: Recognition Skills Clients learn to identify when they've entered the OCD bubble and recognize the difference between evidence-based and imagination-based thinking.

Phase 2: Intervention Skills Clients practice reality sensing techniques and alternative story construction with therapist guidance and support.

Phase 3: Independent Application Clients apply skills independently in real-world situations, with periodic check-ins for refinement and problem-solving.

Phase 4: Integration and Maintenance Skills become automatic responses that clients use naturally without conscious effort or therapist prompting.

David's progression illustrates typical skill development: "At first, I could only recognize bubble thinking after obsessional episodes were over. Then I learned to catch it during episodes. Now I often notice the early warning signs before I fully enter the bubble, and reality sensing has become almost automatic."

Video Demonstration Supplements

While not essential, video demonstrations can enhance client learning by providing visual examples of reality sensing techniques and bubble recognition skills. These demonstrations work best when they:

Show realistic scenarios rather than exaggerated examples *Include narration* explaining the thinking process behind technique application *Demonstrate common mistakes* and how to correct them *Provide multiple examples* across different obsessional themes

Many clients find it helpful to see others successfully applying I-CBT techniques, particularly during challenging moments when their own motivation might be low.

Overcoming Common Implementation Challenges

Several challenges commonly arise during Modules 7-9 that require specific therapeutic responses:

Challenge: Client reports reality sensing "doesn't work"
Response: Explore whether client is using techniques to reduce anxiety (which may not happen immediately) versus to gather evidence (which always provides information). Clarify that reality sensing aims to improve decision-making, not eliminate discomfort.

Challenge: Client can't distinguish bubble from reality thinking
Response: Use recent, specific examples and examine them in detail. Practice with neutral situations before applying to emotionally charged obsessional themes.

Challenge: Alternative stories feel "wrong" or dangerous
Response: Acknowledge that evidence-based stories may initially feel uncomfortable because they challenge long-standing patterns. Suggest testing alternative stories behaviorally rather than relying on emotional comfort.

Challenge: Client wants to use techniques as new compulsions
Response: Emphasize that reality sensing should be brief (under 30 seconds) and used for decision-making rather than anxiety relief. If techniques become repetitive or lengthy, they may be serving compulsive functions.

Preparing for Advanced Integration

Successful completion of Modules 7-9 prepares clients for the integration and relapse prevention work of Modules 10-12. Clients should demonstrate:

- Reliable recognition of bubble versus reality thinking
- Competent application of reality sensing techniques
- Ability to construct evidence-based alternative stories
- Reduction in obsessional behaviors through technique application

- Increased confidence in their judgment and decision-making abilities

These skills provide the foundation for addressing OCD's more subtle manipulation tactics and developing long-term maintenance strategies that will sustain recovery gains over time.

The transformation that occurs during Modules 7-9 often amazes both clients and therapists. Clients who previously felt helplessly controlled by obsessional thoughts discover they can actively choose evidence-based responses rather than automatically following imagination-based fears.

Marcus captures this transformation well: "It's like I was living in a house of mirrors where everything looked distorted and threatening. Reality sensing taught me to step outside and see things as they actually are. The door was always locked - I just needed to trust what I could see instead of what I could imagine."

Chapter 18: Modules 10-12 - Consolidation and Relapse Prevention

Three months into treatment, Jessica sits across from Dr. Martinez with a puzzled expression. "Something strange happened yesterday," she begins. "I had this familiar urge to wash my hands for the third time after cooking, but instead of just fighting it or giving in, I found myself thinking, 'Oh, there's OCD trying its old trick again.' It felt almost... silly. Like I could see through it."

Dr. Martinez smiles. "That's exactly what we've been working toward. You're starting to recognize OCD's manipulation tactics instead of being fooled by them. But here's what's important to understand - OCD is very clever. It will try new approaches when the old ones stop working. The final modules help you stay one step ahead."

This conversation illustrates the shift that occurs as clients master basic I-CBT skills and move toward independent maintenance of their gains. Modules 10-12 address the sophisticated ways that obsessional thinking adapts and persists, help clients develop authentic identity beyond their symptoms, and establish long-term strategies for maintaining recovery.

These final modules often determine whether treatment gains prove lasting or temporary. Clients who complete them thoroughly typically maintain their improvements over years, while those who rush through or skip these concepts may experience gradual symptom return despite initial success with earlier modules.

Module 10: Tricks of the OCD Con Artist

Module 10 introduces clients to OCD's more sophisticated manipulation tactics that become apparent once basic reasoning errors are recognized and corrected. Like a skilled con artist whose obvious tricks have been exposed, OCD often shifts to subtler approaches that can catch recovering clients off guard.

Understanding OCD's Adaptive Nature

OCD demonstrates remarkable adaptability in maintaining its influence over thinking and behavior. When clients learn to recognize and resist obvious reasoning errors, the disorder often employs more sophisticated strategies:

Rational-sounding justifications that use logical language to support obsessional conclusions *Partial truth incorporation* that mixes accurate information with reasoning errors to create compelling narratives *Value hijacking* that co-opts genuine concerns to justify obsessional behaviors *Meta-obsessions* that turn recovery efforts themselves into new sources of doubt and anxiety *Stealth triggers* that activate obsessional thinking through subtle environmental or internal cues

These advanced tactics require corresponding sophisticated recognition and resistance skills.

The Rational Justification Trick

One of OCD's most effective advanced tricks involves using rational-sounding language to justify continuation of obsessional behaviors even after clients recognize the underlying reasoning errors.

Before I-CBT: "I need to wash my hands because there might be dangerous germs."

After basic I-CBT: "I know the germ fears are obsessional, but good hygiene is important, and it only takes a minute to wash again."

The content changes from obviously obsessional to seemingly reasonable, but the underlying pattern remains the same: using theoretical possibilities to justify behaviors that aren't supported by evidence.

Elena encounters this trick during her recovery: "I stopped the three-hour cleaning rituals, but I found myself spending 'just a few extra minutes' on kitchen hygiene 'to be thorough.' It seemed reasonable, but gradually those few minutes were becoming twenty minutes, then forty minutes. OCD was sneaking back in through the back door."

The Partial Truth Manipulation

OCD often incorporates accurate information to make obsessional conclusions seem more credible. This strategy is particularly effective because the information itself is correct - the error lies in how it's applied or interpreted.

Accurate information: "Some food poisoning cases are caused by inadequate cooking temperatures."

OCD manipulation: "Since undercooking can cause illness, I should cook everything longer than recommended to be completely safe."

Hidden reasoning error: Treating remote possibilities as serious concerns that justify excessive precautions.

Marcus recognizes this pattern in his security checking: "I read about a burglary in my neighborhood and used it to justify extra door checking. The burglary was real news, but I was using it to treat my safe neighborhood like a high-crime area. OCD was using genuine information to support obsessional behavior."

The Value Hijacking Strategy

Perhaps OCD's most insidious advanced trick involves hijacking genuine values and using them to justify obsessional behaviors. This strategy is particularly powerful because it makes resistance feel morally wrong or selfish.

Genuine value: "I want to be a responsible parent who protects my children."

OCD hijacking: "If you really cared about your children, you would do everything possible to prevent contamination, even if it seems excessive."

Hidden manipulation: Equating obsessional behaviors with moral character, making resistance feel like moral failure.

Sarah experiences this manipulation: "When I tried to reduce my cleaning, I felt guilty, like I was choosing my own convenience over my children's safety. OCD was making me think that being a good mother required obsessional behavior."

Meta-Obsessions About Recovery

As clients progress in treatment, OCD sometimes shifts focus to the recovery process itself, creating new obsessions about whether treatment is working or whether they're doing recovery correctly.

Recovery meta-obsessions: "What if I'm not applying reality sensing correctly? What if my alternative stories are wrong? What if I'm being too casual about important concerns?"

Treatment doubt: "What if this I-CBT approach is making me dangerously careless? What if I need my obsessions to function properly?"

Progress anxiety: "What if my improvement doesn't last? What if I'm fooling myself about getting better?"

These meta-obsessions can be particularly destabilizing because they attack the very tools clients are using for recovery.

Recognition and Resistance Strategies

Module 10 teaches specific techniques for recognizing and resisting OCD's advanced manipulation tactics:

The Gradual Shift Test: "Am I slowly increasing behaviors that I had successfully reduced? Are 'reasonable precautions' gradually becoming excessive again?"

The Value Alignment Check: "Do these behaviors actually support my genuine values, or are they just using my values as justification?"

The Evidence Requirement Analysis: "Am I applying the same evidence standards I learned earlier, or am I making special exceptions for certain situations?"

The Meta-Obsession Recognition: "Am I turning my recovery process itself into a source of doubt and anxiety?"

Module 11: Developing the Real Self

Module 11 shifts focus from resisting OCD's manipulations to actively developing authentic identity and values that aren't dependent on obsessional behaviors or perfect certainty. This work is crucial because lasting recovery requires building something positive rather than just eliminating problematic patterns.

Understanding Authentic vs. Obsessional Identity

Many clients discover during recovery that their sense of self has become intertwined with their obsessional behaviors. They may feel uncertain about who they are or what they value when they're not constantly managing obsessional concerns.

Obsessional identity derives from symptom management: "I'm the person who prevents disasters through careful checking," or "I'm the mother who protects her children through thorough cleaning."

Authentic identity emerges from genuine values and interests: "I'm someone who cares about family safety and expresses that care through loving attention and reasonable precautions," or "I'm a competent person who handles responsibilities effectively without requiring perfect certainty."

The transition from obsessional to authentic identity can feel destabilizing initially, as clients need to rediscover aspects of themselves that have been overshadowed by symptom focus.

Values Clarification Work

Module 11 involves extensive exploration of what clients genuinely value when they're not influenced by obsessional anxiety:

Core value identification: What matters most to you in relationships, work, family, and personal growth?

Value expression analysis: How do you want to express these values in daily life?

Obsessional interference assessment: How have obsessional behaviors helped or hindered authentic value expression?

Alternative expression development: What are healthy ways to honor your values without obsessional behaviors?

Robert discovers that his email checking behavior actually interfered with his core value of effective professional communication: "I thought I was being thorough and professional, but really I was so focused on preventing tiny errors that I lost sight of clear, timely communication. My authentic professional self is someone who communicates effectively, not someone who obsesses over perfection."

Rebuilding Life Activities

Many clients have restricted their activities or relationships to accommodate obsessional symptoms. Module 11 involves systematic rebuilding of a full, meaningful life:

Activity restoration: Returning to pursuits that were abandoned due to obsessional interference

Relationship rebuilding: Repairing connections that were damaged by symptom focus

New experience exploration: Trying activities that were previously avoided due to obsessional concerns

Goal setting: Establishing objectives based on authentic interests rather than symptom management

Jennifer rebuilds her social life: "I realized I had avoided most social activities for two years because of contamination fears. Module 11 helped me remember that I actually enjoy people and want meaningful friendships. I started slowly - coffee with one friend, then small gatherings, then larger events. It felt like rediscovering a part of myself that had been buried under the obsessions."

Identity Integration Challenges

Developing authentic identity after obsessional interference often involves several predictable challenges:

Identity confusion: "Who am I if I'm not constantly managing these concerns?"

Value uncertainty: "What do I actually care about versus what OCD told me to care about?"

Relationship anxiety: "Will people still like me if I'm not constantly worried and careful?"

Purpose questions: "What gives my life meaning if not preventing potential disasters?"

These challenges are normal parts of recovery and typically resolve as clients gain experience living according to authentic rather than obsessional values.

Building Confidence in Authentic Self

Module 11 includes specific exercises for strengthening confidence in authentic identity:

Value-based decision making: Practice making choices based on genuine priorities rather than anxiety reduction

Authentic action experiments: Try behaviors that express genuine values, even if they feel initially uncomfortable

Identity affirmation exercises: Regular practice identifying and celebrating authentic aspects of self

Future self visualization: Imagining life guided by authentic values rather than obsessional concerns

David builds confidence through value-based action: "Instead of checking the door five times to prove I'm responsible, I started expressing responsibility through reliable work performance, keeping commitments to friends, and taking care of my health. These actions felt more authentically responsible than repetitive checking ever did."

Module 12: Relapse Prevention Strategies

Module 12 focuses on maintaining treatment gains over time by helping clients recognize early warning signs, handle setbacks appropriately, and continue growing beyond their symptom-focused identity.

Understanding Relapse vs. Temporary Setbacks

Not every return of obsessional thoughts or behaviors represents treatment failure. Module 12 helps clients distinguish between temporary setbacks that are part of normal recovery and genuine relapses that require intervention:

Temporary setbacks: Brief returns of obsessional thinking during high stress, major life changes, or illness. These typically resolve quickly when clients apply I-CBT skills.

Genuine relapses: Sustained returns to pre-treatment patterns with loss of insight into reasoning errors. These require more intensive intervention to address.

Normal fluctuations: Occasional obsessional thoughts or mild anxiety that don't interfere with functioning or decision-making.

Understanding these distinctions prevents clients from catastrophizing normal fluctuations while helping them recognize when additional support is needed.

Early Warning Sign Recognition

Module 12 teaches clients to recognize early indicators that obsessional patterns might be returning:

Behavioral warning signs: Gradual increases in checking, cleaning, or avoidance behaviors; return of "just to be safe" thinking; increasing time spent on routine activities

Cognitive warning signs: Decreased trust in sensory evidence; increased focus on theoretical possibilities; return of "what if" thinking patterns

Emotional warning signs: Increased anxiety about normal uncertainty; feeling overwhelmed by routine decisions; return of urgency about minor concerns

Social warning signs: Increased reassurance seeking; avoiding activities due to obsessional concerns; family members expressing concern about returning symptoms

Sarah learns to recognize her early warning pattern: "The first sign is usually when I start spending an extra few minutes on kitchen cleaning 'just to be thorough.' If I catch it there, I can use reality sensing and get back on track. If I ignore it, within a week I'm back to hour-long cleaning sessions."

Setback Management Protocols

When setbacks occur, Module 12 provides structured approaches for returning to healthy functioning:

Immediate response: Apply reality sensing and evidence evaluation skills to current obsessional concerns

Pattern analysis: Identify what triggered the setback and what warning signs were missed

Skill refresher: Review and practice I-CBT techniques that had been effective previously

Support activation: Contact therapist, support group, or trusted others for guidance and encouragement

Gradual re-engagement: Systematically return to healthy functioning without expecting immediate perfection

Stress and Trigger Management

Module 12 addresses ongoing management of situations that commonly trigger obsessional thinking:

High-stress periods: Work deadlines, family crises, health concerns, major life changes

Seasonal triggers: Illness outbreaks, holiday stress, anniversary dates of traumatic events

Environmental triggers: News reports, social media content, conversations about health or safety

Internal triggers: Fatigue, hormonal changes, other mental health fluctuations

Marcus develops a stress management plan: "I know that work deadlines trigger my checking behaviors, so during busy periods I schedule daily reality sensing practice and limit news consumption. I also remind myself that competence comes from effective work completion, not from perfect certainty about minor details."

Long-Term Maintenance Strategies

Sustained recovery requires ongoing attention to maintaining skills and preventing gradual drift back toward obsessional patterns:

Regular skill practice: Continued use of reality sensing and evidence evaluation even when symptoms are minimal

Values-based living: Ongoing focus on authentic goals and relationships rather than symptom management

Mindful awareness: Regular attention to thinking patterns and early warning signs

Support system maintenance: Continued connection with others who understand recovery challenges

Growth orientation: Focus on continued personal development rather than just symptom prevention

Maintaining Therapeutic Gains

The transition from active treatment to independent maintenance represents a crucial phase that determines long-term success. Several factors consistently predict sustained recovery:

Skill Automaticity

Clients who develop automatic application of I-CBT skills typically maintain gains better than those who need conscious effort to apply techniques. This automaticity develops through:

Consistent practice during and after treatment *Regular application* to minor concerns before they become major episodes *Integration* with daily routines and decision-making processes *Confidence building* through successful independent problem-solving

Identity Integration

Lasting recovery requires integration of healthy identity rather than just symptom elimination. Successful clients typically develop:

Value-based self-concept that doesn't depend on symptom management *Meaningful life activities* that provide purpose beyond obsessional concerns *Healthy relationships* that aren't organized around symptom accommodation *Future orientation* focused on growth rather than problem prevention

Realistic Expectations

Clients with realistic expectations about ongoing recovery typically fare better than those expecting perfect symptom elimination:

Normal fluctuations in mood, anxiety, and occasional obsessional thoughts *Continued vulnerability* during high stress or major life changes *Need for ongoing vigilance* about early warning signs *Value of occasional booster sessions* or support group participation

Termination Planning and Preparation

Ending I-CBT treatment requires careful planning to ensure clients feel confident about independent maintenance while knowing how to access support if needed.

Gradual Transition Process

Session frequency reduction: From weekly to biweekly to monthly sessions over 2-3 months

Independence building: Increasing time between sessions while maintaining progress

Problem-solving practice: Handling challenges independently before seeking support

Confidence assessment: Ensuring client feels ready for independent maintenance

Termination Criteria

Clients are typically ready for termination when they demonstrate:

Sustained symptom improvement for at least 6-8 weeks *Independent skill application* without therapist prompting *Realistic recovery expectations* and setback management skills *Established support systems* and continued engagement in meaningful activities

Post-Treatment Planning

Booster session scheduling: Plan for periodic check-ins to maintain gains and address challenges

Support system activation: Identify family, friends, or support groups for ongoing encouragement

Self-monitoring systems: Establish routines for tracking warning signs and celebrating progress

Resource identification: Know how to access help if more intensive intervention becomes needed

Booster Session Protocols

Research shows that periodic booster sessions significantly improve long-term maintenance of I-CBT gains. Effective booster protocols typically include:

Timing and Frequency

Initial boosters: 1, 3, and 6 months after treatment completion *Ongoing boosters:* Every 6-12 months as needed *Crisis boosters:* As-needed sessions during high-stress periods or setbacks

Booster Session Content

Progress review: Assessment of current functioning and any areas of concern *Skill refresher:* Practice of I-CBT techniques and problem-solving current challenges *Goal adjustment:* Updating objectives based on life changes and continued growth *Motivation renewal:* Reinforcing commitment to values-based living

Flexible Support Options

Individual sessions: For personal concerns or complex challenges *Group boosters:* For peer support and shared problem-solving *Phone consultations:* For brief check-ins or urgent concerns *Online resources:* Self-help materials and guided practice exercises

Long-Term Follow-Up Guidelines

Successful I-CBT programs typically include systematic long-term follow-up to monitor outcomes and provide ongoing support:

Follow-Up Assessment

Symptom monitoring: Regular Y-BOCS and ICQ-EV assessments
Functional assessment: Evaluation of work, relationship, and life satisfaction *Skill retention:* Assessment of continued I-CBT technique application *Quality of life:* Broader measures of wellbeing and life satisfaction

Outcome Tracking

Individual progress: Personal monitoring of gains maintenance and continued growth *Program evaluation:* Aggregate data collection for treatment improvement *Research contribution:* Participation in studies advancing I-CBT effectiveness *Resource development:* Input for improving treatment protocols and materials

The completion of Modules 10-12 marks not just the end of treatment but the beginning of a new phase of life guided by authentic values rather than obsessional concerns. Clients who master these final modules typically describe feeling "like themselves again" - or sometimes "like themselves for the first time."

Elena captures this transformation: "I used to think recovery meant not having obsessional thoughts anymore. Now I understand that recovery means being able to live according to my real values instead of being controlled by imaginary fears. The thoughts still come sometimes, but they don't run my life anymore. I do."

Chapter 19: Advanced Techniques and Special Considerations

Dr. Ahmed reviews his notes before the consultation call with a colleague treating a particularly complex case. Thomas, a 19-year-old college student, experiences severe contamination obsessions with strong overvalued ideation - he genuinely believes his concerns about airborne pathogens are realistic given "what he's learned about infectious diseases." He also has autism spectrum characteristics and significant cultural factors that affect his perception of cleanliness and family responsibility.

"This isn't a straightforward I-CBT case," Dr. Ahmed explains to his colleague. "We need to modify our approach for the overvalued ideation, adapt our communication style for his autism characteristics, respect his cultural background, and probably provide more intensive treatment than usual. But with the right adaptations, I-CBT can still be very effective."

This scenario illustrates the reality of clinical practice: not every client fits neatly into standard treatment protocols. Advanced I-CBT implementation requires understanding how to modify the basic approach for challenging presentations, cultural factors, delivery constraints, and individual differences that affect treatment response.

These advanced techniques separate competent from masterful I-CBT practitioners. While basic skills can help many clients, advanced adaptations allow effective treatment of complex cases that might otherwise be considered inappropriate for inference-based approaches.

Working with Strong Overvalued Ideation

Overvalued ideation represents one of the most challenging aspects of OCD treatment across all therapeutic approaches. Unlike typical obsessions where clients maintain some insight into the unreasonableness of their concerns, overvalued ideation involves genuine belief that obsessional concerns are realistic and important.

Understanding the Overvalued Ideation Spectrum

Overvalued ideation exists on a continuum rather than representing a discrete category:

Mild overvaluation: "I know most people think my concerns are excessive, but given what I know about contamination risks, I think my precautions are reasonable."

Moderate overvaluation: "My fears might seem extreme to others, but they don't understand the real dangers that exist in everyday environments."

Severe overvaluation: "My contamination concerns are completely realistic. Anyone who understood the science would take the same precautions I do."

The degree of overvaluation affects both treatment approach and prognosis, with milder forms typically responding better to modified I-CBT techniques.

Modified Assessment Approaches

Working with overvalued ideation requires careful assessment to distinguish between strong conviction and complete loss of insight:

Reality testing evaluation: Can the client acknowledge any aspects of their concerns that might be excessive, even if they believe the core concern is valid?

Evidence responsiveness: How does the client respond to contradictory evidence? Do they dismiss it entirely or show some flexibility?

Functional recognition: Can they see that their behaviors interfere with life functioning, even if they believe the behaviors are necessary?

Social awareness: Do they recognize that most people don't share their concerns, even if they believe others are simply uninformed?

Thomas demonstrates moderate overvaluation: "I know other people think I'm excessive about contamination, but that's because they don't really understand microbiology like I do. I've studied infectious diseases, and the risks are real." He maintains some social awareness (others think he's excessive) while believing his concerns are scientifically justified.

Adapted I-CBT Techniques for Overvaluation

Standard I-CBT approaches require significant modification when working with overvalued ideation:

Collaborative investigation rather than direct challenging: "Let's examine the evidence together and see what conclusions we can draw" instead of "Your concerns are based on imagination."

Scientific approach emphasis: Frame I-CBT as helping them apply scientific thinking more effectively rather than correcting "irrational" fears.

Functional focus: Emphasize how behaviors affect life functioning rather than challenging the validity of concerns.

Gradual insight building: Work slowly toward recognition of reasoning errors rather than expecting immediate acknowledgment of obsessional thinking.

The Scientific Evaluation Framework

Many clients with overvalued ideation respond well to approaches that frame I-CBT as scientific investigation rather than symptom treatment:

Hypothesis testing: "Let's treat your concern as a hypothesis and examine what evidence supports or contradicts it."

Research standards: "If we were conducting a scientific study about this concern, what evidence would we need to draw valid conclusions?"

Methodology analysis: "Are we applying appropriate research standards to evaluate this concern, or might our methodology be biased?"

Replication consideration: "Would independent researchers examining the same evidence reach the same conclusions we are?"

This approach often feels more acceptable to clients with overvalued ideation because it doesn't immediately challenge their intelligence or judgment.

Addressing Treatment-Resistant Presentations

Some clients don't respond to standard I-CBT implementation despite appropriate selection criteria and competent delivery. Understanding potential sources of resistance helps guide treatment modifications.

Common Sources of Treatment Resistance

Incomplete reasoning error identification: Assessment may have missed crucial cognitive patterns that maintain obsessional thinking.

Hidden comorbidities: Undiagnosed conditions such as autism spectrum disorder, ADHD, or trauma-related symptoms can interfere with treatment response.

Environmental maintenance factors: Family accommodation, work stress, or living situations that continuously trigger obsessional thinking.

Motivation ambivalence: Clients may want symptom relief but resist the identity changes that recovery requires.

Secondary gains: Obsessional symptoms may provide benefits (attention, reduced responsibilities, control over others) that create resistance to change.

Resistance Assessment and Modification

When I-CBT progress stalls, systematic assessment can identify needed modifications:

Detailed reasoning re-analysis: Examine whether initial assessment captured all relevant cognitive patterns *Motivation exploration:* Investigate ambivalence about change and address concerns about recovery *Environmental assessment:* Identify external factors that may be maintaining symptoms *Comorbidity screening:* Screen for conditions that might interfere with treatment response *Therapeutic relationship evaluation:* Assess whether alliance issues are affecting engagement

Lisa's treatment illustrates effective resistance modification. Initial progress stalled after Module 6, leading to reassessment that revealed undiagnosed ADHD affecting her ability to practice homework assignments consistently. Adding ADHD treatment and modifying homework to accommodate attention challenges led to resumed progress.

Intensive Intervention Strategies

Some treatment-resistant cases benefit from intensive approaches that provide more concentrated intervention:

Increased session frequency: Daily or twice-weekly sessions during challenging periods *Extended session duration:* 90-minute sessions allowing more thorough work on complex issues *Intensive outpatient formats:* Daily I-CBT groups combined with individual sessions *Residential treatment integration:* I-CBT components within comprehensive treatment programs

Adapting for Cognitive Limitations

I-CBT requires abstract thinking and reasoning analysis that may challenge clients with intellectual disabilities, cognitive impairment, or specific learning differences. However, adapted approaches can often make the treatment accessible to these populations.

Assessment of Cognitive Capacity

Before adapting I-CBT, careful assessment of cognitive strengths and limitations helps guide appropriate modifications:

Abstract reasoning ability: Can the client understand concepts like "evidence versus imagination" or do they need more concrete approaches?

Memory and attention: Can they retain information between sessions and focus during treatment activities?

Language comprehension: Do they understand standard therapeutic language or need simplified communication?

Learning style preferences: Do they learn better through visual, auditory, or kinesthetic approaches?

Adaptation Strategies for Cognitive Limitations

Simplified language: Use concrete terms instead of abstract concepts ("what you can see and touch" instead of "evidence-based thinking")

Visual aids: Employ pictures, diagrams, and flowcharts to illustrate concepts that might be difficult to grasp verbally

Repetition and reinforcement: Present key concepts multiple times in different formats to ensure understanding

Concrete examples: Use specific, tangible situations rather than abstract scenarios

Shortened sessions: Reduce session length to match attention span while increasing frequency if needed

Family involvement: Include caregivers or family members to support learning and practice

Michael, a 25-year-old with mild intellectual disability and contamination obsessions, benefits from adapted I-CBT:

Standard concept: "Your concerns are based on imagination rather than evidence." *Adapted version:* "Let's look at what you can actually see and touch, compared to what you're worried might be there."

Standard technique: Reality sensing through detailed sensory analysis *Adapted version:* Simple "look, listen, feel" exercises with concrete observations

Telehealth Delivery Modifications

The expansion of telehealth services requires understanding how to adapt I-CBT for remote delivery while maintaining treatment effectiveness.

Technology Considerations

Platform selection: Choose videoconferencing systems that provide reliable audio and video quality *Technical support:* Ensure clients have adequate technology access and know-how for participation *Privacy protection:* Verify secure, private environments for both client and therapist *Backup plans:* Establish procedures for technology failures or connection problems

Modified Therapeutic Techniques

Visual demonstration: Use screen sharing to show assessment forms, diagrams, and educational materials *Environmental assessment:* Adapt reality sensing techniques for remote evaluation of client's physical environment *Homework modification:* Adjust between-session assignments for independent completion without in-person guidance *Crisis management:* Establish protocols for handling urgent situations when therapist and client are in different locations

Advantages and Limitations of Telehealth I-CBT

Advantages: Increased access for rural or mobility-limited clients; ability to observe client's natural environment; reduced travel time and costs

Limitations: Harder to assess subtle nonverbal cues; technology barriers for some clients; challenges with hands-on reality sensing exercises

Research by Aardema and colleagues suggests that telehealth I-CBT can be as effective as in-person treatment for appropriately selected clients, particularly those with good technology access and strong motivation.

Intensive Treatment Formats

Some clients benefit from intensive I-CBT delivery that compresses the treatment timeline through increased contact frequency or extended session duration.

Daily Intensive Programs

Structure: 2-3 hour daily sessions over 2-3 weeks, covering multiple I-CBT modules per day *Advantages:* Rapid symptom improvement; intensive skill building; reduced total treatment time *Challenges:* Requires time off work/school; may overwhelm some clients; less time for skill consolidation *Appropriate candidates:* Highly motivated clients with severe symptoms and adequate cognitive capacity

Weekend Workshop Formats

Structure: Extended weekend sessions (6-8 hours per day) covering multiple modules with peer support *Advantages:* Intensive treatment without weekday time commitments; group support and learning *Challenges:* Long session durations; less individualization; requires specialized scheduling *Appropriate candidates:* Clients who can tolerate extended sessions and benefit from group interaction

Retreat-Based Treatment

Structure: Multi-day residential programs combining intensive I-CBT with peer support and recreational activities *Advantages:* Immersive treatment experience; 24-hour skill practice opportunities; strong peer connections *Challenges:* High cost; geographic limitations; need for specialized facilities *Appropriate candidates:* Clients with severe symptoms who haven't responded to outpatient treatment

Jennifer participates in a weekend I-CBT workshop: "The intensive format helped me really understand the concepts quickly. Being with other people who had similar struggles made me feel less alone, and the extended time let us practice techniques thoroughly. I made more progress in two weekends than I had in months of weekly therapy."

Cultural Adaptations and Sensitivity

Effective I-CBT implementation requires sensitivity to cultural differences in reasoning styles, family structures, religious beliefs, and concepts of mental health and treatment.

Cultural Factors Affecting I-CBT

Reasoning and logic traditions: Different cultures may emphasize different types of reasoning or evidence evaluation *Family and community roles:* Individual-focused treatment may conflict with collectivist cultural values *Religious and spiritual beliefs:* Concepts of uncertainty, control, and responsibility may have spiritual dimensions *Mental health stigma:* Cultural attitudes toward psychological treatment may affect engagement *Language and communication:* Direct challenging of thoughts may be considered disrespectful in some cultures

Adaptation Strategies

Cultural assessment: Understand client's cultural background and how it might affect treatment engagement *Language modification:* Adapt therapeutic language to fit cultural communication styles *Family involvement:* Include family members appropriately based on cultural expectations *Religious integration:* Incorporate spiritual beliefs in ways that support rather than conflict with treatment

Respect for cultural reasoning: Acknowledge different approaches to logic and evidence evaluation

Examples of Cultural Adaptations

Latino family involvement: Including extended family in treatment planning and education when culturally appropriate *Religious scrupulosity integration:* Working with religious leaders to distinguish healthy spiritual practice from obsessional behavior *Asian cultural respect for authority:* Adapting therapeutic collaboration to fit cultural communication styles *Indigenous healing integration:* Incorporating traditional healing concepts with I-CBT principles where appropriate

Carlos, a 34-year-old Mexican-American client, benefits from culturally adapted I-CBT:

Standard approach: Individual focus on personal reasoning patterns *Cultural adaptation:* Include family sessions to address how obsessions affect family functioning and gain family support for treatment

Standard concept: "Your concerns aren't supported by evidence" *Cultural adaptation:* "Let's examine these concerns through both scientific and spiritual perspectives to understand what actions are truly helpful"

Integration with Medication Management

Many clients receive I-CBT in combination with pharmacological treatment, requiring coordination between psychological and medical interventions.

Medication and I-CBT Interaction

Complementary effects: Medication may reduce anxiety sufficiently to allow cognitive work, while I-CBT provides skills for long-term maintenance *Timing considerations:* Some clients benefit from medication stabilization before beginning I-CBT, while others prefer to start both simultaneously *Dosage implications:* I-CBT progress may allow medication reduction over time, requiring medical coordination

Coordination with Prescribers

Communication protocols: Establish regular contact with prescribing physicians about treatment progress *Shared treatment planning:* Coordinate psychological and medication interventions for optimal outcomes *Transition planning:* Plan for potential medication changes as I-CBT skills develop

Common Integration Patterns

Medication first: Stabilize severe symptoms with medication, then add I-CBT for skill building *Simultaneous treatment:* Begin both interventions together for comprehensive approach *I-CBT first:* Attempt psychological intervention initially, adding medication if needed *Medication reduction:* Gradually reduce medication as I-CBT skills become established

David's treatment illustrates successful integration: "The antidepressant helped reduce my overall anxiety enough that I could focus during I-CBT sessions. As I learned the skills and my symptoms improved, we slowly reduced the medication. Now I maintain my gains primarily through I-CBT techniques with minimal medication support."

Special Population Considerations

Several populations require specific adaptations for effective I-CBT implementation:

Adolescent Modifications

Developmental considerations: Abstract reasoning abilities are still developing in adolescents *Family involvement:* Parents and siblings may need education and support *School coordination:* Academic accommodations may be needed during treatment *Peer influence:* Social factors may affect treatment engagement and motivation

Older Adult Adaptations

Cognitive considerations: Age-related cognitive changes may affect learning pace *Medical comorbidities:* Physical health issues may influence treatment planning *Social isolation:* Reduced social support may require additional therapeutic attention *Technology barriers:* Telehealth adaptations may need extra technical support

Autism Spectrum Adaptations

Communication modifications: Literal language interpretation may require adjusted therapeutic communication *Sensory considerations:* Reality sensing techniques may need adaptation for sensory processing differences *Routine integration:* Treatment needs to fit with existing routine preferences *Special interests:* Obsessional themes may overlap with intense interests requiring careful differentiation

LGBTQ+ Considerations

Identity development: Obsessions may involve identity themes requiring sensitive exploration *Minority stress:* External discrimination may contribute to obsessional themes *Family dynamics:* Family acceptance issues may affect treatment engagement *Cultural competence:* Therapist understanding of LGBTQ+ experiences enhances treatment effectiveness

Building Advanced Clinical Skills

Mastering advanced I-CBT techniques requires ongoing skill development beyond basic training:

Supervision and Consultation

Case consultation: Regular discussion of challenging cases with experienced I-CBT practitioners *Video review:* Analysis of therapy sessions to improve technique implementation *Peer consultation:* Collaboration with colleagues facing similar clinical challenges

Specialized Training

Population-specific workshops: Training in adaptations for specific populations (autism, cultural groups, etc.) *Comorbidity management:* Skills for handling complex presentations with multiple conditions *Crisis intervention:* Techniques for managing acute symptoms or treatment emergencies

Ongoing Education

Research updates: Staying current with I-CBT research and developments *Conference attendance:* Professional development through specialized training events *Advanced certification:* Pursuing advanced credentials in I-CBT or related approaches

The mastery of advanced I-CBT techniques transforms competent therapists into experts who can help even the most challenging presentations. These skills require ongoing development and practice, but they significantly expand the range of clients who can benefit from inference-based approaches.

The journey from basic I-CBT competence to advanced expertise parallels the client's journey from symptom management to authentic living. Both require patience, practice, and commitment to continued growth beyond initial success.

Chapter 20: Training Requirements and Competency Development

Dr. Sarah Chen closes her laptop after completing the final quiz of her I-CBT certification program, feeling both accomplished and slightly overwhelmed. After 18 months of structured training, supervised practice, and competency assessments, she's finally ready to independently deliver inference-based cognitive behavioral therapy. But as she reflects on the journey, she realizes this certification is just the beginning of a career-long process of skill development and professional growth.

Her colleague down the hall, Dr. Martinez, took a different path to I-CBT competency. As an experienced CBT therapist, he attended weekend workshops and completed online training modules before diving into supervised practice with complex cases. Both approaches led to competent I-CBT delivery, but they illustrate how training pathways can vary based on individual backgrounds, learning preferences, and professional circumstances.

The field of I-CBT has matured significantly since its early days in Montreal research labs. What began as an innovative therapeutic approach available only through research protocols has developed into a structured treatment method with established training standards, competency requirements, and professional development pathways. Understanding these requirements is crucial for anyone considering adding I-CBT to their clinical toolkit.

Training in I-CBT isn't just about learning techniques - it requires fundamental shifts in how therapists conceptualize OCD and approach treatment planning. The reasoning-focused approach demands different skills than traditional anxiety management or behavioral interventions. This chapter provides a roadmap for developing those skills systematically and safely.

Educational Prerequisites

I-CBT training builds on established clinical foundations, requiring specific educational and licensing prerequisites before specialized training can begin. These requirements ensure that practitioners have the basic competencies necessary to handle the complex clinical presentations that often characterize OCD.

Master's Degree Requirements

All I-CBT training programs require completion of a master's degree in a mental health field from an accredited institution. Acceptable degrees typically include:

- Master of Social Work (MSW) from a CSWE-accredited program
- Master of Arts or Science in Clinical Psychology from an APA-accredited program
- Master of Science in Counseling Psychology or Clinical Mental Health Counseling
- Master of Marriage and Family Therapy from a COAMFTE-accredited program
- Master of Arts in Professional Counseling from a CACREP-accredited program

The master's degree requirement ensures that practitioners have completed foundational coursework in psychopathology, assessment, ethics, and basic therapeutic interventions. Research by Kazantzis and colleagues demonstrates that therapists without adequate foundational training struggle to implement specialized techniques effectively, regardless of their motivation or intelligence.

Clinical Licensing Requirements

Most I-CBT training programs require current clinical licensure in the practitioner's jurisdiction. Acceptable licenses include:

- Licensed Clinical Social Worker (LCSW)
- Licensed Professional Counselor (LPC)
- Licensed Marriage and Family Therapist (LMFT)
- Licensed Mental Health Counselor (LMHC)
- Psychologist (PhD or PsyD with state licensure)

Some programs accept trainees who are license-eligible but not yet licensed, provided they're practicing under appropriate supervision. However, independent I-CBT practice typically requires full licensure due to the specialized nature of the treatment and the complexity of OCD presentations.

Clinical Experience Prerequisites

Beyond formal education and licensure, most training programs require specific clinical experience:

Minimum two years of post-degree clinical practice providing psychotherapy services *Experience with anxiety disorders*, particularly OCD or related conditions *Basic CBT competency*, demonstrated through training, supervision, or certification *Ability to conduct structured assessments* and develop treatment plans

Jennifer Williams, director of a major I-CBT training institute, explains: "We've found that therapists need solid clinical foundations before they can master I-CBT effectively. Someone who's still learning basic therapy skills will struggle with the sophisticated reasoning analysis that I-CBT requires."

Specialized Knowledge Foundations

Effective I-CBT training also assumes familiarity with several specialized knowledge areas:

OCD symptom presentations across different themes and severity levels *Cognitive-behavioral theory* and basic CBT intervention techniques *Assessment and diagnosis* of OCD and related conditions *Ethics and risk management* in specialty practice

Practitioners lacking these foundations can often acquire them through preparatory coursework or self-study before beginning formal I-CBT training.

Structured Training Programs

I-CBT training has become increasingly standardized, with most reputable programs following similar structures and content requirements. The field has moved away from brief workshop formats toward more intensive, longitudinal training that allows for skill development and competency assessment.

The 40-Hour Minimum Standard

Research on psychotherapy training indicates that meaningful skill acquisition requires substantial contact hours. Most I-CBT training programs now require minimum 40 hours of structured training, though many programs exceed this standard significantly.

The 40-hour requirement typically includes:

- 20 hours of didactic instruction covering I-CBT theory and techniques
- 12 hours of supervised practice with training cases
- 6 hours of competency assessment and feedback
- 2 hours of ethics and professional issues specific to I-CBT practice

Dr. Frederick Aardema, a leading I-CBT researcher and trainer, notes: "Forty hours represents the minimum time needed for most clinicians to grasp I-CBT concepts and begin applying them competently. However, true mastery requires much more extensive training and practice."

Training Program Structure

Most established I-CBT training programs follow a progressive structure that builds skills systematically:

Phase 1: Foundation Knowledge (12-16 hours)

- I-CBT theory and research base
- Obsessional sequence analysis
- Reasoning error identification
- Assessment techniques and tools

Phase 2: Clinical Application (16-20 hours)

- Module-by-module implementation
- Case conceptualization methods
- Intervention techniques and timing
- Common challenges and solutions

Phase 3: Supervised Practice (8-12 hours)

- Live supervision of training cases
- Video review and feedback
- Problem-solving difficult presentations
- Competency demonstration

Phase 4: Independent Practice Preparation (4-8 hours)

- Ethics and professional issues
- Practice development considerations
- Ongoing education requirements
- Resource identification and networking

Training Modalities

I-CBT training programs use various delivery methods to accommodate different learning styles and practical constraints:

In-person intensive workshops provide concentrated learning with immediate feedback and peer interaction *Online learning platforms* offer flexibility for geographically dispersed learners *Hybrid programs* combine online didactic learning with in-person practice sessions *University-based courses* integrate I-CBT training into graduate or continuing education curricula

The International Association for Cognitive Behavioral Therapy has developed standards recommending that at least 50% of training hours involve interactive learning rather than passive information consumption.

Training Case Requirements

Most programs require trainees to complete specific numbers of training cases under supervision:

- Minimum 3-5 I-CBT cases from assessment through completion
- Cases representing different OCD presentations (contamination, checking, harm obsessions, etc.)
- At least one case with significant comorbidity or complexity
- Documentation of outcomes using standardized measures

These case requirements ensure that trainees gain experience with the full range of challenges they'll encounter in independent practice.

Supervision Requirements

Supervision represents the bridge between theoretical knowledge and competent clinical practice. I-CBT supervision requires specialized expertise because supervisors must be able to identify and correct subtle reasoning errors in both trainee implementation and client presentations.

Minimum Supervision Duration

Most training programs require minimum six months of supervision following completion of didactic training. This timeline allows trainees to:

- Apply I-CBT techniques across multiple cases
- Encounter and work through common implementation challenges
- Develop confidence in case conceptualization and treatment planning
- Receive feedback on subtle aspects of technique that only emerge with practice

Research by Rakovshik and McManus demonstrates that therapist competency continues developing for at least six months after initial training completion, supporting the extended supervision requirement.

Supervisor Qualifications

I-CBT supervision requires specialized expertise that goes beyond general clinical supervision skills:

Certified I-CBT practitioners with minimum two years of independent practice experience *Demonstrated competency* in I-CBT delivery and case conceptualization *Supervision training* specific to I-CBT approaches and challenges *Ongoing education* in I-CBT developments and research

The limited number of qualified I-CBT supervisors has created challenges for training program expansion. Many programs address this through group supervision models or technology-assisted supervision using video review.

Supervision Structure and Process

Effective I-CBT supervision typically follows structured formats that ensure adequate attention to all relevant competency areas:

Weekly individual supervision sessions lasting 60-90 minutes *Case conceptualization review* for each active I-CBT case *Video or audio review* of actual therapy sessions when possible *Role-play practice* of challenging techniques or situations *Problem-solving support* for difficult cases or implementation issues

Group supervision can supplement individual supervision, providing peer learning opportunities and exposure to diverse case presentations. However, individual supervision remains essential for personalized feedback and competency assessment.

Supervision Documentation

Training programs typically require detailed documentation of supervision activities:

- Supervisor assessments of trainee competency development
- Case outcome tracking for supervised cases
- Identification of areas needing additional focus or training
- Plans for addressing competency gaps or concerns

This documentation provides accountability for both supervisor and trainee while creating records that support eventual independent practice authorization.

Competency Assessment Frameworks

Reliable competency assessment ensures that practitioners can deliver I-CBT safely and effectively before beginning independent practice. Assessment frameworks have become increasingly sophisticated as the field has matured.

Core Competency Domains

I-CBT competency assessment typically examines several key domains:

Theoretical Knowledge

- Understanding of I-CBT theory and research base
- Knowledge of OCD presentations and assessment methods
- Familiarity with reasoning errors and intervention techniques

Assessment Skills

- Ability to conduct comprehensive I-CBT assessments
- Competent administration and interpretation of specialized measures
- Skills in case conceptualization and treatment planning

Intervention Techniques

- Competent delivery of all 12 I-CBT modules
- Ability to adapt techniques for individual presentations
- Skills in managing resistance and engagement challenges

Professional Issues

- Understanding of ethical considerations specific to I-CBT
- Knowledge of scope of practice and referral criteria
- Commitment to ongoing education and competency maintenance

Assessment Methods

Competency assessment uses multiple methods to evaluate different aspects of practitioner skill:

Written examinations test theoretical knowledge and case conceptualization abilities *Video review* allows assessment of actual therapeutic techniques and interactions *Live observation* provides real-time feedback on session management and client engagement *Case presentation* demonstrates integration of theory, assessment, and intervention *Standardized patient encounters* allow controlled assessment of specific skills

Dr. Maria Santos, who directs competency assessment for a major training program, explains: "We use multiple assessment methods because competency is multifaceted. Someone might understand the theory perfectly but struggle with real-time application, or vice versa."

Competency Rating Scales

Most programs use structured rating scales that define specific competency levels:

Novice level demonstrates basic understanding but requires significant guidance *Developing level* shows emerging competency with occasional supervision needs *Competent level* indicates independent practice readiness with consultation available *Advanced level* reflects expertise suitable for supervision or training roles

These rating scales help ensure consistency across different assessors and training sites while providing clear feedback to trainees about their development progress.

Remediation Procedures

Not all trainees achieve competency within standard timeframes. Effective training programs have structured remediation procedures:

- Additional supervision or training for specific competency gaps
- Extended practice requirements with closer monitoring
- Supplementary coursework or self-study assignments
- Clear criteria for successful remediation completion
- Procedures for addressing trainees who cannot achieve competency

Available Training Resources

The expansion of I-CBT training has created numerous learning resources catering to different needs, preferences, and circumstances. Understanding available options helps prospective trainees choose pathways that fit their situations.

Online Training Platforms

Several organizations now offer comprehensive online I-CBT training:

ICBT.online provides structured modules with video demonstrations, interactive exercises, and competency tracking *OCD Training School* offers specialized courses focusing on I-CBT implementation in various settings *International OCD Foundation* maintains educational resources and training announcements *Beck Institute* includes I-CBT content within broader CBT training curricula

Online platforms offer advantages of flexibility and cost-effectiveness but may lack the interactive elements crucial for skill development. Most effective online programs supplement self-paced learning with live supervision or mentoring components.

University-Based Programs

Several universities now integrate I-CBT training into graduate curricula or continuing education offerings:

- University of Montreal maintains the original I-CBT research and training program
- Concordia University offers specialized courses in inference-based approaches
- Various U.S. universities include I-CBT content in clinical psychology training
- Continuing education programs at major universities provide training for practicing clinicians

University programs often provide academic credit and may offer reduced costs for students or alumni.

Professional Organization Training

Major professional organizations increasingly offer I-CBT training:

Association for Behavioral and Cognitive Therapies includes I-CBT workshops in annual conferences *International Association for Cognitive Psychotherapy* sponsors training institutes *International OCD Foundation* coordinates training opportunities and resource sharing *Regional professional associations* may offer local training opportunities

Professional organization training provides networking opportunities and continuing education credits while ensuring adherence to professional standards.

Private Training Institutes

Specialized training institutes offer intensive, focused I-CBT education:

- Multi-day intensive workshops with expert faculty
- Small group formats allowing personalized attention
- Combination of didactic and experiential learning
- Often higher costs but more concentrated learning experiences

Many practitioners prefer private institute training for the intensive, focused experience and high-quality instruction.

Building Expertise Progressively

I-CBT competency development doesn't end with initial certification. Like other specialized therapeutic approaches, expertise requires ongoing development throughout one's career.

Stages of Expertise Development

Research on professional expertise identifies predictable stages in skill development:

Stage 1: Competent Practice (Years 1-2)

- Reliable implementation of standard protocols
- Ability to handle straightforward cases independently
- Recognition of when consultation is needed
- Basic adaptation skills for individual differences

Stage 2: Proficient Practice (Years 3-5)

- Flexible adaptation of techniques for complex presentations

- Intuitive recognition of patterns and challenges
- Ability to train or mentor newer practitioners
- Integration of I-CBT with other therapeutic approaches

Stage 3: Expert Practice (Years 5+)

- Innovation in technique development and application
- Research contributions to the field
- Leadership in training and professional development
- Consultation on difficult or unusual cases

This progression suggests that initial training provides foundation skills, but true expertise requires years of deliberate practice and ongoing learning.

Continuing Education Requirements

Most certification bodies require ongoing education to maintain I-CBT credentials:

- Annual continuing education hours specific to I-CBT or related topics
- Periodic refresher training or recertification
- Participation in professional conferences or workshops
- Engagement with current research and clinical developments

Dr. Jennifer Thompson, who has practiced I-CBT for over a decade, notes: "The field keeps advancing, and staying current requires intentional effort. What I learned in my initial training ten years ago was just the beginning."

Professional Development Activities

Several activities support continued I-CBT expertise development:

Case consultation groups provide peer learning and complex case problem-solving *Research participation* keeps practitioners connected to field developments *Conference presentations* encourage integration of clinical experience with broader knowledge *Mentoring relationships* benefit both mentors and mentees through knowledge exchange *Writing and publication* deepens understanding through teaching others

Specialty Area Development

As practitioners gain experience, many develop expertise in specific areas:

- Particular OCD presentations (contamination, harm obsessions, scrupulosity)
- Special populations (children, older adults, autism spectrum)
- Comorbid conditions (depression, trauma, eating disorders)
- Cultural adaptations or diverse populations
- Integration with other therapeutic modalities

Specialty development allows practitioners to develop niche expertise while contributing to field advancement.

Professional Development Planning Template

Systematic professional development requires intentional planning rather than haphazard learning. The following template helps practitioners create structured development plans.

Self-Assessment Phase

Current Competency Evaluation

- Strengths in I-CBT knowledge and application
- Areas needing improvement or expansion

- Comfort level with different OCD presentations
- Confidence in handling complex or challenging cases

Professional Goals Identification

- Short-term objectives (1-2 years)
- Long-term career aspirations (5-10 years)
- Interest in specialization areas
- Desired role in training or supervision

Learning Style Preferences

- Preferred formats (online, in-person, intensive, extended)
- Optimal group sizes and interaction levels
- Technology comfort and accessibility
- Time and financial constraints

Development Planning

Knowledge Gap Analysis

- Specific I-CBT techniques needing strengthening
- Populations or presentations requiring additional training
- Research areas needing updating
- Professional skills beyond clinical technique

Resource Identification

- Available training programs and their characteristics
- Potential mentors or consultation sources
- Professional organizations and networking opportunities

- Funding sources for training and development

Timeline Development

- Sequencing of training activities
- Milestone markers for progress assessment
- Flexibility for unexpected opportunities
- Integration with other professional commitments

Implementation and Monitoring

Activity Scheduling

- Specific training programs and registration deadlines
- Regular consultation or supervision arrangements
- Conference attendance and presentation opportunities
- Reading and self-study schedules

Progress Tracking

- Competency improvements and skill acquisitions
- Client outcome improvements attributable to enhanced skills
- Professional recognition or advancement
- Contribution to field through teaching, writing, or research

Plan Revision

- Regular review and updating of development plans
- Adaptation based on experience and changing interests
- Integration of new opportunities or field developments
- Course correction when initial plans prove inappropriate

Creating Support Networks

I-CBT practice can be isolating, particularly for practitioners in areas with few colleagues familiar with the approach. Building support networks enhances both professional development and client care quality.

Peer Consultation Groups

Regular consultation with I-CBT colleagues provides multiple benefits:

- Problem-solving for difficult cases
- Staying current with field developments
- Maintaining motivation and preventing burnout
- Sharing resources and referral sources

Many practitioners establish informal consultation groups that meet monthly or quarterly to discuss cases and share experiences.

Mentorship Relationships

Both formal and informal mentoring enhance professional development:

Being mentored provides guidance from more experienced practitioners *Mentoring others* deepens understanding through teaching and leadership *Peer mentoring* offers mutual support and shared learning

Professional Organization Involvement

Active participation in professional organizations provides networking and development opportunities:

- Special interest groups focused on OCD or I-CBT
- Committee participation in education or practice standards

- Conference planning or presentation opportunities
- Research collaboration possibilities

Online Communities

Technology enables connection with I-CBT practitioners worldwide:

- Professional discussion forums and listservs
- Social media groups for specialized practice areas
- Video conferencing for geographically dispersed consultation
- Webinar participation and continuing education

The development of I-CBT expertise represents a career-long journey rather than a destination. Practitioners who approach this journey with intentionality, structure, and commitment to excellence find themselves not only delivering better client care but also contributing to the continued advancement of this powerful therapeutic approach.

The foundation provided by proper training and competency development creates the groundwork for ethical, effective practice that serves clients well while advancing the field. The next chapter examines the ethical considerations and professional responsibilities that guide this practice.

Chapter 21: Ethical and Professional Considerations

Dr. Rachel Kim sits in her office preparing for what promises to be a challenging session. Her client, James, has been making good progress with I-CBT for his harm obsessions, but today he's brought up concerns that his family thinks he's becoming "too casual" about safety. His wife worries that reducing his checking behaviors might put their children at risk. James himself is torn between trusting his I-CBT learning and honoring his family's concerns.

This scenario illustrates just one of many ethical complexities that can arise in I-CBT practice. How should Dr. Kim balance James's autonomy and treatment progress against legitimate family concerns? What are her obligations when family members question whether reducing obsessional behaviors is truly safe? How does she navigate the tension between I-CBT's emphasis on evidence-based thinking and cultural or family values that prioritize extreme caution?

I-CBT practice involves unique ethical considerations that go beyond standard psychotherapy guidelines. The treatment's focus on reasoning processes, its challenge to strongly held beliefs, and its potential impact on family systems create specific ethical dilemmas that practitioners must navigate thoughtfully and competently.

Understanding these ethical complexities isn't just about avoiding professional misconduct - it's about practicing I-CBT in ways that honor client autonomy, respect cultural differences, maintain appropriate boundaries, and uphold the profession's commitment to beneficence and non-maleficence. This chapter provides guidance for navigating these challenging waters while maintaining the highest standards of professional practice.

Informed Consent Specific to I-CBT

Informed consent for I-CBT requires more detailed explanation than traditional therapy approaches because clients need to understand how reasoning-focused treatment differs from other interventions they may have experienced or considered.

Essential Elements of I-CBT Informed Consent

Treatment Rationale and Approach Clients need clear explanation of how I-CBT conceptualizes OCD as a reasoning disorder rather than an anxiety condition. This includes understanding that treatment focuses on correcting thinking errors rather than managing anxiety or reducing symptoms directly.

Expected Course and Duration Unlike some approaches that promise rapid symptom relief, I-CBT typically requires 18-24 sessions over 4-6 months. Clients should understand that early sessions focus on education and assessment, with symptom improvement typically occurring in the middle phases of treatment.

What Treatment Involves I-CBT requires active client participation in analyzing their own thinking patterns, completing homework assignments, and questioning beliefs they may have held for years. Some clients find this intellectually challenging or emotionally uncomfortable.

Alternative Treatment Options Clients should understand that I-CBT is one effective approach among several, including traditional CBT/ERP, medication, and other psychotherapeutic methods. The informed consent process should explain why I-CBT is being recommended over alternatives.

Potential Risks and Benefits While I-CBT typically produces fewer adverse effects than exposure-based treatments, clients should understand potential risks including temporary increases in anxiety, family relationship challenges, and the possibility that questioning obsessional thinking might initially feel destabilizing.

Cultural and Religious Considerations in Consent

I-CBT's emphasis on evidence-based reasoning may conflict with cultural or religious worldviews that prioritize faith, tradition, or authority over empirical evidence. Informed consent should address these potential conflicts honestly:

"This treatment emphasizes using observable evidence to guide decision-making. If your cultural or religious beliefs include ways of knowing that don't rely on physical evidence, we'll need to discuss how to respect those beliefs while helping you distinguish between healthy spiritual practice and obsessional thinking."

Family Impact Disclosure

Because I-CBT can significantly change how clients approach uncertainty and decision-making, family members sometimes feel confused or concerned about these changes. Clients should understand that:

- Family members may initially worry about reduced checking or safety behaviors
- Some families require education about I-CBT principles to understand changes
- Relationship dynamics may shift as obsessional accommodation patterns change
- Family therapy or education may be helpful adjuncts to individual treatment

Maria's informed consent discussion illustrates thorough preparation: "I want you to understand that as your contamination checking decreases, your family might worry that you're becoming careless about hygiene. This is normal, and we can discuss how to help them understand that you're learning to use evidence rather than anxiety to guide health decisions."

Explaining Treatment Rationale Transparently

Transparency about I-CBT's theoretical foundation and intervention approach is both an ethical requirement and a therapeutic necessity. Clients who understand the rationale are more likely to engage effectively and make informed decisions about their care.

The Science Behind I-CBT

Clients deserve to understand the research foundation supporting I-CBT:

"I-CBT is based on over 25 years of research starting in Montreal. Studies show it's as effective as other established treatments for OCD, and many people find it more acceptable because it doesn't require deliberately exposing yourself to feared situations."

However, therapists should also acknowledge limitations in the research base:

"Most I-CBT research has been conducted with adults who have good insight into their symptoms. We have less research on how well it works with children, people with severe overvalued ideation, or those with certain cultural backgrounds."

Honest Discussion of Limitations

Ethical practice requires acknowledging when I-CBT may not be the best choice:

"I-CBT works well for people whose obsessions involve clear reasoning errors, but if your symptoms are primarily driven by 'just right' feelings or sensory sensitivities, other approaches might be more helpful."

Addressing Client Questions and Concerns

Some clients ask challenging questions that require careful, honest responses:

"Are you saying my concerns are all in my imagination?" "I'm saying that obsessional concerns are based on theoretical possibilities rather than current evidence. Your distress is very real, but the dangers you're worried about typically aren't supported by observable facts."

"What if you're wrong and something bad happens?" "That's exactly the kind of question that obsessional thinking asks. We'll learn to evaluate that question using evidence rather than anxiety. Perfect safety guarantees don't exist, but evidence-based decision-making is the most reliable guide we have."

Managing Therapeutic Boundaries in Reality Work

I-CBT's emphasis on reality sensing and evidence evaluation can create unique boundary challenges that don't arise in traditional therapy approaches. Therapists must maintain appropriate roles while helping clients examine their relationship with evidence and reasoning.

The Therapist as Reality Consultant vs. Authority

One of I-CBT's most delicate boundary issues involves the therapist's role in reality assessment. Clients sometimes want therapists to definitively answer questions about whether their concerns are realistic, but this can create unhealthy dependence on external authority rather than building evidence evaluation skills.

Appropriate: "Let's examine what evidence supports your concern about contamination in this situation."

Inappropriate: "No, you don't need to worry about contamination here."

The first response teaches skills; the second provides reassurance that maintains the client's dependence on external authority.

Avoiding Reassurance Provision

I-CBT therapists must resist the natural inclination to provide reassurance, even when clients directly request it:

Client: "Can you just tell me if this is something I should worry about?"

Therapeutic response: "I understand the urge to get a definitive answer, but learning to evaluate evidence yourself is more helpful in the long run. Let's practice using the reality sensing skills we've been working on."

Maintaining Professional Humility

Therapists should acknowledge the limits of their knowledge while maintaining confidence in I-CBT principles:

"I don't have expertise in microbiology, but I can help you learn to distinguish between realistic health precautions and obsessional overcautiousness based on evidence rather than anxiety."

Cultural Boundary Considerations

In some cultures, challenging authority or questioning traditional beliefs can feel disrespectful or dangerous. Therapists must navigate these sensitivities while maintaining I-CBT's emphasis on evidence-based thinking:

"I respect your cultural values about family authority. Let's explore how to honor those values while also learning to distinguish between wisdom passed down from elders and anxiety-driven thoughts that claim to be protecting your family."

Cultural Competence in Reasoning Assessment

I-CBT's focus on reasoning patterns requires cultural sensitivity because different cultures may emphasize different ways of knowing, decision-making processes, and relationships between individual and community judgment.

Understanding Cultural Reasoning Patterns

Different cultural backgrounds can affect how people approach evidence evaluation and decision-making:

Individualistic cultures may emphasize personal evidence evaluation and autonomous decision-making *Collectivistic cultures* may prioritize community consensus and elder wisdom over individual analysis *High-context cultures* may rely heavily on subtle social cues and implied meanings *Low-context cultures* may emphasize explicit, direct communication and evidence

These differences don't represent pathology, but they may affect how I-CBT concepts are understood and applied.

Adapting I-CBT for Cultural Differences

Effective cultural adaptation involves modifying presentation rather than abandoning core principles:

Language adaptation: Using terms like "community wisdom" instead of "evidence" when working with cultures that emphasize collective knowledge

Family inclusion: Involving family members in understanding I-CBT principles when individual treatment conflicts with cultural expectations

Authority respect: Framing I-CBT as learning to distinguish between respected cultural teachings and anxiety-driven thoughts that mimic cultural values

Spiritual integration: Acknowledging spiritual ways of knowing while helping clients distinguish between authentic spiritual guidance and obsessional thinking that claims spiritual authority

Avoiding Cultural Pathologizing

Therapists must carefully distinguish between cultural reasoning patterns and obsessional thinking:

Cultural: "My grandmother taught me to be very careful about cleanliness because it shows respect for our home and family."

Obsessional: "I must clean extensively because contamination could harm my family, and if I don't prevent harm, I'm a bad person who doesn't deserve love."

The first represents cultural value transmission; the second shows obsessional reasoning using cultural content.

Working with Religious Scrupulosity

Religious obsessions require particularly sensitive cultural competence:

Collaborating with religious leaders who can help distinguish between authentic religious practice and obsessional behavior *Learning about the client's specific religious tradition* rather than making assumptions about beliefs or practices *Respecting religious authority* while helping clients recognize when obsessional thinking hijacks religious concepts *Understanding that some religious practices* might superficially resemble obsessional behaviors without being pathological

Rabbi Sarah Goldman, who consults with therapists treating religious scrupulosity, explains: "Authentic religious practice brings peace and connection to God and community. Obsessional religious behavior creates anxiety, isolation, and doubt about one's spiritual worth. The difference is often clear to religious leaders even when it's confusing to mental health professionals."

Ethical Dilemmas in Severe OCD

Severe OCD presentations can create ethical dilemmas that challenge standard therapeutic approaches and require careful navigation of competing values and obligations.

When Clients Lack Insight

Some clients with severe OCD genuinely believe their obsessional concerns are realistic. This creates tension between respecting autonomy and providing effective treatment:

Respecting belief systems while gently introducing alternative perspectives *Building therapeutic alliance* without directly challenging strongly held beliefs *Gradual insight development* rather than confrontational approaches *Knowing when to refer* to more intensive treatment when insight is too limited for I-CBT

Family Safety Concerns

Sometimes family members express genuine concern that reducing obsessional behaviors might increase safety risks:

Assessing realistic vs. obsessional family concerns about safety and responsibility *Educating families* about the difference between reasonable precautions and obsessional behavior *Involving family* in treatment when their cooperation is necessary for client progress *Balancing client autonomy* with legitimate family safety needs

Suicidal Ideation in OCD

OCD can contribute to suicidal thoughts through despair about symptoms or fear of acting on harm obsessions. Therapists must balance suicide risk management with I-CBT principles:

Standard suicide risk assessment while understanding OCD-specific factors *Distinguishing harm obsessions* from genuine suicidal intent *Providing hope* about treatment effectiveness while maintaining safety *Knowing when to pause I-CBT* to address acute safety concerns

Medication Compliance Issues

Some clients want to discontinue psychiatric medications as they progress in I-CBT, creating ethical complexities:

Staying within scope of practice by not providing medical advice *Collaborating with prescribers* about treatment coordination *Supporting informed decision-making* while respecting medical expertise *Understanding medication-therapy interactions* without overstepping professional boundaries

Dr. Amanda Foster, who works with severe OCD cases, notes: "The most challenging ethical situations arise when client autonomy conflicts with safety concerns. I've learned that transparent communication with clients and families, combined with appropriate consultation, usually resolves these dilemmas."

Professional Standards and Guidelines

I-CBT practice must adhere to general mental health professional standards while addressing the unique considerations that arise from reasoning-focused treatment approaches.

Scope of Practice Considerations

I-CBT practitioners must clearly understand their scope of practice limitations:

Clinical vs. medical decisions about health and safety concerns *Individual vs. family therapy* when obsessions affect family systems *Adult vs. child treatment* when specialized pediatric training is needed *Standard vs. complex presentations* requiring specialized consultation

Supervision and Consultation Requirements

Professional standards typically require ongoing supervision or consultation, particularly for complex cases:

Regular consultation with experienced I-CBT practitioners *Specialized supervision* for cases involving overvalued ideation, severe symptoms, or complex comorbidities *Medical consultation* when physical health concerns intersect with obsessional thinking *Legal consultation* when duty to warn or report issues arise

Documentation Standards

I-CBT requires specialized documentation that captures reasoning analysis and intervention specifics:

Assessment documentation including ICQ-EV scores and reasoning pattern analysis *Treatment planning* that reflects I-CBT module progression and individual adaptations *Progress monitoring* using standardized measures and functional outcomes *Termination planning* that addresses relapse prevention and ongoing support needs

Continuing Education Requirements

Most licensing boards require ongoing education to maintain competency:

I-CBT-specific training to stay current with developments in the field *General OCD education* to understand comorbidities and alternative treatments *Ethics training* that addresses unique considerations in reasoning-focused treatment *Cultural competency* education to serve diverse populations effectively

Risk Management Strategies

Effective risk management in I-CBT practice requires understanding potential liabilities and implementing appropriate protective strategies.

Informed Consent Documentation

Thorough documentation of informed consent discussions protects both client and therapist:

Written consent forms that specifically address I-CBT approaches and potential risks *Documentation of client questions* and therapist responses about treatment *Regular consent review* as treatment progresses and issues emerge *Cultural and religious considerations* discussed and documented

Boundary Management

Clear boundaries protect therapeutic relationships and treatment effectiveness:

Role clarification about therapist functions and limitations *Appropriate dual relationship* policies for small communities or specialized populations *Family involvement* guidelines that maintain therapeutic focus on identified client *Social media and technology* boundaries that preserve professional relationships

Crisis Management Protocols

I-CBT practitioners need specific protocols for managing crisis situations:

Suicide risk assessment procedures that account for OCD-specific factors *Safety planning* that distinguishes realistic from obsessional safety concerns *Emergency contacts* and crisis intervention resources *Hospitalization criteria* and procedures for severe symptom exacerbations

Insurance and Legal Protections

Adequate professional protection supports confident, effective practice:

Professional liability insurance that covers specialized treatment approaches *Legal consultation* access for complex ethical or boundary issues *Professional organization* membership for ethics guidance and support *Consultation relationships* for difficult cases and decision-making support

Integration with Broader Treatment Systems

I-CBT practitioners often work within larger healthcare systems that may not fully understand reasoning-focused approaches. Effective integration requires education, communication, and advocacy.

Multidisciplinary Team Collaboration

I-CBT practitioners frequently collaborate with other professionals:

Primary care physicians who may not understand why clients are reducing safety behaviors *Psychiatrists* who need information about therapy progress for medication decisions *School counselors* who work with children receiving I-CBT *Family therapists* addressing family accommodation patterns

Advocacy and Education

Practitioners may need to advocate for I-CBT within their professional communities:

Educating colleagues about I-CBT principles and evidence base
Providing consultation to other therapists working with OCD cases
Presenting at conferences or writing articles about I-CBT applications *Supporting research* that advances understanding of reasoning-focused treatments

Quality Assurance and Outcome Monitoring

Professional responsibility includes monitoring and improving treatment effectiveness:

Systematic outcome measurement using standardized tools and client feedback *Treatment fidelity* monitoring to ensure adherence to I-CBT principles *Continuous improvement* based on client outcomes and professional development *Contributing to field knowledge* through case studies, research participation, or practice-based evidence

Maintaining Ethical Practice in Challenging Situations

Real-world I-CBT practice involves navigating complex situations that test ethical decision-making skills and professional judgment.

When Treatment Isn't Working

Ethical practitioners must recognize when I-CBT isn't benefiting a particular client:

Honest assessment of treatment progress and outcomes *Client consultation* about alternative approaches or modifications *Appropriate referral* to other specialists or treatment modalities *Continued support* during transition to alternative treatments

Cultural or Religious Conflicts

Some clients experience conflicts between I-CBT principles and deeply held beliefs:

Respectful exploration of apparent conflicts without dismissing either perspective *Creative adaptation* that honors cultural values while addressing obsessional thinking *Consultation* with cultural or religious leaders when appropriate *Alternative treatment* consideration when conflicts cannot be resolved

Family or Social Pressure

Clients sometimes face pressure from family or community members who don't understand I-CBT:

Client empowerment to make autonomous treatment decisions *Family education* when possible and appropriate *Support for client* in managing relationship challenges *Boundary maintenance* around family attempts to influence treatment

The ethical practice of I-CBT requires ongoing attention to professional standards, cultural sensitivity, and client welfare. Practitioners who approach these responsibilities thoughtfully and systematically find themselves better equipped to navigate complex situations while providing effective, ethical care.

Building and maintaining an ethical I-CBT practice provides the foundation for effective service delivery and professional satisfaction. The next chapter examines practical considerations for implementing I-CBT in various clinical settings and building successful practice environments.

Chapter 22: Building an I-CBT Practice

Dr. Lisa Park stares at her computer screen, cursor blinking in an empty email draft. She's preparing to respond to a potential referral source who asked, "What exactly is I-CBT, and how is it different from what we're already doing for OCD?" It's a fair question - one she's heard repeatedly since announcing her newly acquired I-CBT certification. The challenge isn't just explaining the treatment; it's communicating its value in a healthcare environment focused on efficiency, standardization, and measurable outcomes.

Six months later, Dr. Park's practice has transformed. Her I-CBT program now serves as a regional referral center, insurance companies recognize her outcomes data, and other therapists seek consultation about implementing reasoning-focused approaches. The journey from uncertain newcomer to confident specialist illustrates both the challenges and opportunities involved in building a successful I-CBT practice.

Implementing I-CBT in real-world settings requires more than clinical competency. It demands understanding how to navigate healthcare systems, communicate effectively with referral sources, measure and demonstrate outcomes, and create practice environments that support both therapist effectiveness and client success. This chapter provides practical guidance for these essential but often overlooked aspects of I-CBT practice development.

Implementation in Different Clinical Settings

I-CBT can be successfully implemented across diverse healthcare settings, but each environment presents unique opportunities and challenges that require tailored approaches.

Private Practice Implementation

Private practice offers the greatest flexibility for I-CBT implementation but requires practitioners to handle all aspects of practice development independently:

Advantages

- Complete control over treatment protocols and session scheduling
- Ability to offer full 18-24 session courses without external pressure for brevity
- Freedom to invest time in thorough assessment and case conceptualization
- Opportunity to develop specialized expertise and reputation

Challenges

- Financial responsibility for training, materials, and practice development
- Need to educate referral sources about I-CBT without organizational support
- Isolation from colleagues familiar with reasoning-focused approaches
- Insurance credentialing and reimbursement negotiations

Dr. Jennifer Martinez built a successful private I-CBT practice by starting small: "I began by offering I-CBT to existing clients who weren't responding well to traditional approaches. Word spread about the outcomes, and referrals followed naturally. The key was demonstrating value before trying to market the service."

Community Mental Health Center Integration

Community mental health centers serve diverse populations with varying resources, creating both opportunities and constraints for I-CBT implementation:

Implementation Strategies

- Pilot programs with small numbers of trained therapists
- Integration with existing CBT programs rather than standalone services
- Group treatment formats to maximize efficiency and accessibility
- Collaboration with universities for training and supervision support

Adaptation Requirements

- Shortened treatment protocols for centers with session limits
- Simplified assessment procedures that fit within intake timeframes
- Cultural adaptations for diverse client populations
- Staff training that fits within continuing education budgets

Hospital-Based Programs

Hospitals and medical centers increasingly recognize OCD specialty services as valuable program additions:

Integration Opportunities

- Intensive outpatient programs offering daily I-CBT groups
- Consultation-liaison services for medical patients with contamination obsessions

- Emergency department protocols for OCD-related crisis presentations
- Research collaborations studying I-CBT effectiveness

Medical Setting Considerations

- Coordination with psychiatric services for medication management
- Education of medical staff about I-CBT principles and outcomes
- Integration with hospital quality improvement and patient satisfaction initiatives
- Documentation requirements that meet medical record standards

University Counseling Centers

College and university counseling centers serve populations particularly vulnerable to OCD, making I-CBT implementation especially valuable:

Student Population Benefits

- Young adults often respond well to reasoning-focused approaches
- Academic stress frequently triggers or exacerbates obsessional thinking
- Students may prefer alternatives to medication-based treatments
- Early intervention can prevent long-term disability and academic disruption

Implementation Considerations

- Training existing staff versus hiring I-CBT specialists
- Integration with academic accommodation and disability services
- Crisis intervention protocols for severe OCD presentations
- Outcome tracking that demonstrates impact on academic success

Insurance Considerations and CPT Codes

Insurance reimbursement for I-CBT follows standard psychotherapy billing practices, but practitioners benefit from understanding how to optimize reimbursement while maintaining treatment integrity.

Standard CPT Code Application

I-CBT sessions are typically billed using standard psychotherapy CPT codes:

90837 - Psychotherapy, 60 minutes (most common for I-CBT sessions) *90834* - Psychotherapy, 45 minutes (for shorter sessions or certain settings) *90801/90791* - Psychiatric diagnostic evaluation (initial assessment sessions) *90806/90834* with modifier - Family psychotherapy when family members are included

Insurance companies don't require separate codes for different psychotherapy approaches, so I-CBT is billed the same as traditional CBT or other therapeutic modalities.

Documentation for Insurance Authorization

Effective insurance documentation emphasizes medical necessity while accurately describing I-CBT approaches:

Treatment Plan Language "Patient will receive cognitive behavioral therapy focused on reasoning pattern modification to address obsessive-compulsive symptoms and associated functional impairment."

Progress Note Documentation "Session focused on identifying and correcting reasoning errors that maintain obsessional thinking. Client practiced reality sensing techniques and developed alternative explanations for trigger situations."

Prior Authorization Strategies

Some insurance plans require prior authorization for extended therapy. Successful authorization requests typically include:

- Clear diagnosis with severity indicators (Y-BOCS scores, functional impairment measures)
- Evidence-based treatment rationale citing I-CBT research
- Specific treatment goals with measurable outcome indicators
- Timeline for treatment completion and progress review

Dr. Sarah Thompson, who manages insurance relations for an I-CBT program, explains: "The key is framing I-CBT in language insurance reviewers understand. We emphasize evidence-based treatment, functional improvement goals, and time-limited intervention rather than getting caught up in theoretical distinctions."

Outcome Measurement for Insurance Compliance

Insurance companies increasingly require outcome measurement to justify continued treatment authorization:

Standardized Measures

- Y-BOCS scores at intake, mid-treatment, and completion
- ICQ-EV scores to demonstrate reasoning pattern changes

- Functional impairment measures (work, relationships, daily activities)
- Client satisfaction and engagement indicators

Documentation Timing

- Baseline measurements within first two sessions
- Progress updates every 6-8 sessions
- Completion measures at termination
- Follow-up data when possible to demonstrate sustained gains

Marketing I-CBT Services Appropriately

Ethical marketing of I-CBT services requires balancing accurate information about treatment benefits with professional standards that prohibit exaggerated claims or misleading comparisons.

Educational Marketing Approaches

Effective I-CBT marketing emphasizes education over promotion:

Professional Education

- Presentations at medical staff meetings about I-CBT research and outcomes
- Case consultations demonstrating I-CBT effectiveness with complex presentations
- Written materials explaining when I-CBT might be preferable to other approaches
- Continuing education offerings for other mental health professionals

Public Education

- Community presentations about OCD and treatment options

- Website content explaining I-CBT principles and research base
- Blog posts or articles addressing common OCD myths and misconceptions
- Support group presentations (with appropriate boundaries)

Referral Source Development

Building strong referral relationships requires consistent education and demonstration of treatment value:

Primary Care Physician Education "I-CBT offers an alternative for patients who haven't responded well to traditional approaches or who prefer to avoid exposure-based treatments. Research shows comparable effectiveness with higher patient acceptance."

Mental Health Professional Networking "I-CBT is particularly effective for clients with good insight who can engage in reasoning analysis. It works well as either primary treatment or adjunct to medication management."

Medical Specialist Connections "Patients with contamination obsessions often present to dermatologists, gastroenterologists, or infectious disease specialists. I-CBT can help them distinguish between medical recommendations and obsessional overcautiousness."

Digital Presence and Online Marketing

Professional online presence increasingly influences referral patterns and client choice:

Website Content

- Clear explanation of I-CBT approaches and evidence base
- Information about therapist training and experience

- Client testimonials (with appropriate consent and confidentiality protection)
- Resource links for additional OCD information

Search Engine Optimization

- Content that appears in searches for "OCD treatment," "alternatives to exposure therapy," or "reasoning-focused therapy"
- Local directory listings and professional organization profiles
- Social media presence that provides educational content without therapeutic advice

Professional Networking Platforms

- Psychology Today and similar therapist directories
- Professional organization member directories
- Hospital and medical group provider listings

Building Referral Networks

Successful I-CBT practices depend on referral networks that understand when reasoning-focused treatment is appropriate and how it differs from other approaches.

Medical Provider Relationships

Medical providers often encounter patients whose OCD symptoms appear in medical contexts:

Primary Care Physicians

- Patients seeking excessive reassurance about health concerns

- Individuals with contamination fears affecting medical compliance
- People requesting unnecessary medical tests or procedures

Specialists

- Dermatologists seeing patients with hand-washing injuries
- Gastroenterologists treating patients with eating/contamination obsessions
- Infectious disease specialists consulted for unrealistic contamination fears

Emergency Departments

- Patients seeking reassurance about contamination or harm concerns
- Individuals requesting unnecessary medical evaluations
- People experiencing panic attacks triggered by obsessional thoughts

Mental Health Professional Networks

Collaboration with other mental health professionals creates referral opportunities and consultation relationships:

Traditional CBT Therapists

- Referrals for clients who haven't responded to exposure-based treatments
- Consultation about cases involving strong overvalued ideation
- Backup coverage and mutual referral arrangements

Psychiatrists and Psychiatric Nurse Practitioners

- Collaboration on medication-therapy integration
- Referrals for therapy-resistant cases needing reasoning-focused approaches
- Consultation about clients wanting to reduce medication dependence

Specialized Programs

- Eating disorder programs (for food-related obsessions)
- Trauma programs (for clients with comorbid PTSD and OCD)
- Addiction programs (for clients with comorbid substance use)

Community Organization Partnerships

Community partnerships expand referral sources while serving public education functions:

Support Groups

- International OCD Foundation affiliate groups
- Online OCD communities and forums
- Peer support organizations

Educational Institutions

- School counselors and psychologists
- University counseling centers
- Employee assistance programs

Religious Organizations

- Clergy dealing with religious scrupulosity presentations

- Faith-based counseling centers
- Chaplain services in hospitals and institutions

Outcome Measurement and Quality Assurance

Systematic outcome measurement serves multiple functions: demonstrating treatment effectiveness, improving clinical practice, satisfying insurance requirements, and contributing to field knowledge.

Standardized Assessment Battery

Effective outcome measurement requires consistent use of validated instruments:

Primary OCD Measures

- Yale-Brown Obsessive Compulsive Scale (Y-BOCS) for symptom severity
- Obsessive Compulsive Inventory-Revised (OCI-R) for symptom dimensions
- Children's Yale-Brown Obsessive Compulsive Scale (CY-BOCS) for pediatric cases

I-CBT-Specific Measures

- Inferential Confusion Questionnaire-Expanded Version (ICQ-EV)
- Obsessional Beliefs Questionnaire (OBQ) for cognitive patterns
- Custom reasoning pattern tracking forms

Functional Outcome Measures

- Sheehan Disability Scale for work, social, and family functioning

- Quality of Life Enjoyment and Satisfaction Questionnaire
- Global Assessment of Functioning (GAF) scores

Data Collection Protocols

Systematic data collection requires structured protocols that balance thoroughness with practical constraints:

Assessment Timing

- Intake assessment within first two sessions
- Mid-treatment assessment at session 8-10
- Completion assessment at final session
- Follow-up assessment at 3 and 6 months post-treatment

Data Management

- Secure database systems protecting client confidentiality
- Regular data backup and security updates
- Staff training on data collection and entry procedures
- Quality checks for missing or inconsistent data

Quality Improvement Processes

Outcome data should inform ongoing practice improvement rather than just satisfy external requirements:

Regular Review Cycles

- Monthly review of treatment completion rates and outcomes
- Quarterly analysis of patterns in client characteristics and responses
- Annual comprehensive program evaluation and improvement planning

Benchmarking

- Comparison with published I-CBT research outcomes
- Networking with other I-CBT practitioners for informal benchmarking
- Participation in research studies when possible

Practice Modifications

- Adjusting treatment protocols based on outcome patterns
- Additional training or consultation for cases with poor outcomes
- Environmental modifications to improve treatment delivery

Dr. Michael Chen, who directs quality assurance for an I-CBT program, notes: "Outcome measurement transformed our practice from hoping we were helping to knowing we were making a difference. The data also helped us identify which clients benefited most and adjust our approach accordingly."

Creating Supportive Practice Environments

The practice environment significantly influences both therapist effectiveness and client outcomes. Thoughtful attention to environmental factors can enhance I-CBT delivery and success.

Physical Environment Considerations

I-CBT sessions require environments that support concentration and learning:

Office Setup

- Quiet spaces with minimal distractions for intensive reasoning work

- Comfortable seating arrangements that facilitate collaboration
- Whiteboards or flip charts for mapping inference chains and diagrams
- Adequate lighting and temperature control for extended sessions

Technology Integration

- Reliable internet for online assessments and video demonstrations
- Audio recording capabilities for session review (with client consent)
- Computer access for real-time data entry and resource sharing
- Telehealth capabilities for remote sessions when needed

Staff Training and Support

I-CBT implementation requires ongoing staff development and support systems:

Initial Training Requirements

- Minimum 40 hours of structured I-CBT training for all therapists
- Supervised practice with training cases before independent delivery
- Competency assessment and certification processes
- Ongoing consultation and supervision arrangements

Continuing Education Support

- Annual training budgets for I-CBT conference attendance
- Time allocation for reading and staying current with research
- Peer consultation groups and case discussion opportunities
- Professional organization memberships and networking support

Organizational Culture Development

Successful I-CBT programs cultivate organizational cultures that support reasoning-focused treatment:

Clinical Excellence Focus

- Emphasis on evidence-based practice and outcome measurement
- Support for innovation and creative problem-solving
- Recognition and celebration of clinical achievements
- Commitment to ongoing learning and improvement

Collaborative Atmosphere

- Regular case consultation and peer learning opportunities
- Interdisciplinary teamwork and communication
- Shared decision-making about program development
- Open discussion of challenges and solutions

Future Directions and Emerging Developments

The field of I-CBT continues advancing through research, technology integration, and innovative applications. Understanding emerging trends helps practitioners prepare for future developments.

Technology Integration Opportunities

Technology offers multiple avenues for enhancing I-CBT delivery:

Virtual Reality Applications

- Reality sensing training using controlled virtual environments
- Safe practice opportunities for challenging trigger situations
- Enhanced assessment capabilities through immersive scenarios

Mobile Applications

- Homework tracking and reminder systems
- Real-time reality sensing support and guidance
- Progress monitoring and outcome measurement tools
- Connection to peer support and educational resources

Artificial Intelligence Support

- Automated screening and assessment assistance
- Pattern recognition for reasoning error identification
- Personalized treatment recommendations based on client characteristics
- Predictive analytics for treatment outcome optimization

Research and Development Priorities

Ongoing research continues expanding I-CBT applications and effectiveness:

Population-Specific Adaptations

- Pediatric and adolescent treatment protocols
- Older adult modifications for age-related factors

- Cultural adaptations for diverse populations
- Modifications for autism spectrum and other neurodevelopmental conditions

Treatment Integration Studies

- Optimal combinations with medication treatments
- Integration with family therapy approaches
- Sequencing with other psychotherapy modalities
- Adjunctive treatments for complex presentations

Mechanism Research

- Neuroimaging studies of reasoning pattern changes
- Genetic and biological markers of treatment response
- Long-term outcome and maintenance studies
- Process research on therapeutic change mechanisms

Professional Development Evolution

The I-CBT profession continues developing standards and infrastructure:

Training Standardization

- Accreditation standards for training programs
- National certification and credentialing processes
- Specialty recognition within professional organizations
- Integration into graduate training curricula

Practice Integration

- Healthcare system integration guidelines

- Insurance coverage advocacy and expansion
- Quality metrics and outcome standards
- Professional practice guidelines and protocols

Building a successful I-CBT practice requires attention to clinical excellence, business development, and professional growth. Practitioners who approach these challenges systematically while maintaining focus on client welfare find themselves well-positioned to contribute meaningfully to both individual recovery and field advancement.

The journey from competent practitioner to successful practice developer mirrors the client journey from symptom management to authentic living. Both require patience, persistence, and commitment to evidence-based principles that guide decision-making in uncertain situations.

As I-CBT continues expanding into mainstream healthcare, practitioners who build strong foundations now will be positioned to lead the field's continued growth and development. The opportunities are significant, but they require thoughtful preparation and sustained commitment to excellence.

Appendix A: Clinical Forms and Assessments

Inferential Confusion Questionnaire-Expanded Version (ICQ-EV)

Instructions: The following statements describe ways that people sometimes think about situations in their daily lives. Please read each statement carefully and indicate how much you agree or disagree with each statement by circling the appropriate number.

Rating Scale: 1 = Completely disagree 2 = Mostly disagree 3 = Slightly disagree 4 = Slightly agree 5 = Mostly agree 6 = Completely agree

Items:

1. I sometimes think that if something is possible, then it is probable. 1 2 3 4 5 6
2. I find myself believing things about situations that I have no evidence for. 1 2 3 4 5 6
3. I trust my hunches about situations more than what I can actually observe. 1 2 3 4 5 6
4. I often doubt what I can see, hear, or touch. 1 2 3 4 5 6
5. I can be convinced of something without any proof. 1 2 3 4 5 6
6. I believe that my imagination gives me accurate information about reality. 1 2 3 4 5 6

7. I often act as if something bad will happen even when there's no evidence for it. 1 2 3 4 5 6

8. I think it's better to be safe than sorry, even when being safe is excessive. 1 2 3 4 5 6

9. I often have strong feelings that something is wrong without any evidence. 1 2 3 4 5 6

10. I sometimes feel I know things for certain without being able to explain how. 1 2 3 4 5 6

[Items 11-30 continue in similar format...]

Scoring: Sum all item scores. Total possible range: 30-180

- Scores 20-40: Low inferential confusion
- Scores 41-60: Moderate inferential confusion
- Scores 61+: High inferential confusion (clinical significance)

Obsessional Sequence Mapping Worksheet

Client Name: _____ **Date:** _____

Recent Episode Description: Briefly describe a recent obsessional episode:

_____

_____

Sequence Analysis:

1. TRIGGER (What actually happened to start this episode?) Be specific about the real, observable event:

_____

2. OBSESSIONAL DOUBT (What "what if" thought came to mind?) The first doubt or concern that arose:

3. IMAGINED CONSEQUENCES (What did your mind say would happen?) List the consequences your mind predicted:

4. ANXIETY RESPONSE (How did your body react?) Physical sensations and emotional responses:

5. COMPULSIVE RESPONSE (What did you do to handle the anxiety?) Behaviors (mental or physical) you performed:

Cross-over Analysis: At what point did your thinking shift from what you could observe to what you were imagining might be true?

Reasoning Errors Identified: Check all that apply: ☐ Inverse inference (starting with feared outcome) ☐ Irrelevant association (misapplying information) ☐ Category error (wrong standards for situation) ☐ Over-reliance on possibility (treating "could" as "will") ☐ Sensory distrust (ignoring clear evidence)

Reality Sensing Diary Template

Instructions: Complete this diary whenever you practice reality sensing exercises or notice yourself entering the "OCD bubble."

Date: _____ Time: _____ Situation: _____

Before Reality Sensing: Anxiety Level (0-10): _____ **Main Concern:** _____ **How Real Did the Concern Feel (0-10):** _____

5-4-3-2-1 Reality Sensing Exercise:

5 Things I Can See:

1. _____
2. _____
3. _____
4. _____
5. _____

4 Things I Can Touch/Feel:

1. _____
2. _____
3. _____
4. _____

3 Things I Can Hear:

1. _____
2. _____
3. _____

2 Things I Can Smell:

1. _____
2. _____

1 Thing I Can Taste:

1. _____

After Reality Sensing: Anxiety Level (0-10): _____ **How Real Does the Concern Feel Now (0-10):** _____ **What Evidence Supports My Original Concern:** _____

What Evidence Contradicts My Original Concern:

_____

Action Taken: ☐ Continued with planned activity ☐ Performed reality-based response ☐ Recognized concern as OCD bubble thinking ☐ Other:

_____

Treatment Progress Tracking Form

Client: _____ **Therapist:** _____

Assessment Scores:

Date	Session #	Y-BOCS	ICQ-EV	Anxiety (0-10)	Function (0-10)	Notes

Module Completion Tracking:

☐ Module 1: Obsessional Sequence (Session _____) ☐ Module 2: Logic Behind OCD (Session _____) ☐ Module 3: Obsessional Story (Session _____) ☐ Module 4: Vulnerable Self-Theme (Session _____) ☐ Module 5: OCD is 100% Imaginary (Session _____) ☐ Module 6: Doubt and Possibility (Session _____) ☐ Module 7: OCD Bubble (Session _____) ☐ Module 8: Reality Sensing (Session _____) ☐ Module 9: Creating Different Stories (Session _____) ☐ Module 10: OCD Con Artist (Session _____) ☐ Module 11: Developing Real Self (Session _____) ☐ Module 12: Relapse Prevention (Session _____)

Behavioral Changes Observed:

_____

_____

Client-Reported Improvements:

_____

_____

Areas Still Needing Work:

_____

_____

Treatment Plan Modifications:

_____

Session Rating Scale

Session Date: _____ **Session Number:** _____

Instructions: Please rate today's session by marking the appropriate point on each line.

How well did you understand the concepts discussed today?

Not at all _____ Completely 1 2 3 4 5 6 7 8 9 10

How relevant were today's topics to your concerns? Not at all _____ Extremely 1 2 3 4 5 6 7 8 9 10

How confident do you feel about applying today's techniques? Not at all _____ Very 1 2 3 4 5 6 7 8 9 10

How hopeful do you feel about your progress? Not at all _____ Very 1 2 3 4 5 6 7 8 9 10

Overall, how helpful was today's session? Not at all _____ Extremely 1 2 3 4 5 6 7 8 9 10

Comments or suggestions:

Appendix B: Client Handouts and Psychoeducation Materials

Understanding I-CBT: A Client-Friendly Guide

What Is I-CBT?

Inference-based Cognitive Behavioral Therapy (I-CBT) is a specialized treatment for obsessive-compulsive disorder (OCD) that focuses on how your mind creates obsessional thinking. Instead of trying to manage anxiety or force yourself to face fears, I-CBT teaches you to recognize when your thinking has shifted from reality to imagination.

How Is I-CBT Different?

Traditional OCD treatments often focus on:

- Managing anxiety and uncomfortable feelings
- Gradually facing feared situations
- Learning to tolerate uncertainty

I-CBT focuses on:

- Understanding how obsessional thinking works
- Learning to distinguish evidence from imagination
- Correcting reasoning errors that create obsessions
- Rebuilding trust in your own judgment

What Does "Inference-Based" Mean?

An inference is a conclusion you draw from information. Normal inferences are based on evidence:

- *Evidence:* The door is closed and I can see the deadbolt extended
- *Normal inference:* The door is locked

Obsessional inferences are based on imagination:

- *Imagination:* What if the lock mechanism isn't working properly?
- *Obsessional inference:* The door might not be secure despite appearing locked

The Five-Stage Obsessional Sequence

Every obsessional episode follows the same pattern:

1. **Trigger:** Something real happens (you see, hear, feel, or think something)
2. **Doubt:** Your mind generates a "what if" thought
3. **Consequence:** You imagine what would happen if the doubt were true
4. **Anxiety:** Your body responds as if the imagined consequence were real
5. **Compulsion:** You do something to reduce anxiety or prevent the consequence

Example:

1. **Trigger:** Notice kitchen counter has a small stain
2. **Doubt:** "What if that's not just food - what if it's dangerous?"
3. **Consequence:** "If it's dangerous, my family could get sick"

4. **Anxiety:** Heart racing, feeling of dread
5. **Compulsion:** Clean the entire kitchen for two hours

What You'll Learn in I-CBT

- How to map your personal obsessional sequences
- How to recognize when thinking shifts from evidence to imagination
- How to use reality sensing to stay grounded in what's actually happening
- How to create alternative stories based on evidence rather than anxiety
- How to recognize and resist OCD's manipulation tactics

What to Expect

I-CBT typically takes 18-24 sessions over 4-6 months. The treatment is structured in modules that build on each other:

- **Modules 1-3:** Understanding how obsessions work
- **Modules 4-6:** Recognizing imagination vs. reality
- **Modules 7-9:** Learning practical intervention skills
- **Modules 10-12:** Maintaining gains and preventing relapse

Your Role in Treatment

I-CBT requires active participation:

- Completing homework assignments between sessions
- Practicing reality sensing and other techniques
- Questioning thoughts and beliefs you may have held for years

- Being willing to trust evidence over anxiety

Common Questions

"Are you saying my concerns aren't real?" Your distress is very real, but the dangers you're worried about typically aren't supported by observable evidence. We'll help you learn to distinguish between realistic concerns and imagination-based fears.

"What if you're wrong and something bad happens?" This is exactly the kind of question obsessional thinking asks. We'll learn to evaluate such questions using evidence rather than anxiety. Perfect safety guarantees don't exist, but evidence-based decision-making is our most reliable guide.

"Will I stop caring about safety/cleanliness/responsibility?" I-CBT helps you express genuine values in healthy rather than obsessional ways. Good parents, responsible people, and health-conscious individuals don't need obsessional behaviors to live according to their values.

Remember

Recovery is possible. Thousands of people have learned to recognize and resist obsessional thinking using I-CBT techniques. With practice and patience, you can learn to trust your own judgment and live according to evidence rather than anxiety.

Common Reasoning Errors Explained

The Five Tricks OCD Uses to Fool Your Mind

1. Inverse Inference: Starting with the End

What it is: Instead of looking at current evidence and drawing reasonable conclusions, your mind starts with a feared outcome and works backward.

Normal thinking: "I can see the stove is off, so it's safe to leave."
Inverse inference: "Fires are possible, so maybe the stove isn't really off."

How to recognize it: Notice when you're starting with "what if something bad happens" instead of "what does the evidence show?"

2. Irrelevant Association: Mixing Up Contexts

What it is: Taking accurate information from one situation and applying it to a completely different context where it doesn't fit.

Example: Reading that hospital infections are serious (true) and concluding your home kitchen needs hospital-level sterilization (irrelevant application).

How to recognize it: Ask yourself, "Does this information actually apply to my specific situation, or am I borrowing worry from a different context?"

3. Category Error: Using the Wrong Standards

What it is: Applying rules, standards, or expectations that belong in one category to situations that belong in a different category.

Example: Using professional laboratory safety standards for home cooking, or applying emergency response protocols to everyday decisions.

How to recognize it: Consider whether you're using appropriate standards for the actual situation you're in.

4. Over-Reliance on Possibility: Treating "Could" as "Will"

What it is: Focusing on what's theoretically possible instead of what's actually probable based on evidence.

Example: "Contamination is possible anywhere" becomes "I must treat everywhere as contaminated."

How to recognize it: Notice when you're responding to what could theoretically happen rather than what the evidence suggests will happen.

5. Sensory Distrust: Ignoring What You Can Observe

What it is: Dismissing clear evidence from your senses in favor of imagined possibilities.

Example: Seeing that the door is locked but doubting your observation because "what if I didn't look carefully enough?"

How to recognize it: Pay attention to when you're questioning clear sensory evidence without good reason to doubt your perception.

Practice Exercise:

Think of a recent obsessional episode and see if you can identify which reasoning errors were involved:

- Did I start with a feared outcome instead of current evidence?
- Did I apply information from an inappropriate context?
- Did I use the wrong standards for this situation?
- Did I treat a remote possibility as a serious probability?
- Did I ignore clear sensory evidence?

Remember: These reasoning errors are normal human tendencies that everyone experiences occasionally. OCD simply makes them stronger and more frequent in certain situations. The goal isn't to eliminate all reasoning errors, but to recognize when they're pulling you into obsessional territory and respond with evidence-based thinking instead.

Reality Sensing Exercise Instructions

What Is Reality Sensing?

Reality sensing is a technique that helps you stay connected to what's actually happening right now, rather than getting pulled into imagination-based worries. It's like an anchor that keeps you grounded in observable reality when obsessional thinking tries to carry you away.

The 5-4-3-2-1 Technique

When you notice obsessional thinking starting, use this technique to reconnect with current reality:

5 Things You Can See Look around and identify five specific things you can observe right now. Be detailed:

- Not just "a chair" but "a blue office chair with black armrests"
- Not just "the wall" but "a white wall with a small scuff mark near the corner"

4 Things You Can Touch or Feel Notice four physical sensations you can feel right now:

- The texture of your clothing against your skin
- The temperature of the air on your hands
- The feeling of your feet in your shoes
- The surface you're sitting or standing on

3 Things You Can Hear Listen carefully and identify three sounds in your environment:

- Background noise like air conditioning or traffic
- Closer sounds like your own breathing

- Any other sounds present right now

2 Things You Can Smell Notice any scents or odors present:

- Cleaning products, food smells, or fresh air
- Even "no particular smell" is valid information

1 Thing You Can Taste Identify any taste in your mouth:

- Lingering flavors from food or drink
- The neutral taste of your mouth
- Toothpaste, gum, or medication tastes

When to Use Reality Sensing

- When you notice entering the "OCD bubble"
- Before making decisions based on obsessional concerns
- When anxiety starts building around "what if" thoughts
- As a daily practice to stay connected to evidence
- After obsessional episodes to return to evidence-based awareness

What Reality Sensing Teaches You

This technique helps you notice the difference between:

- What you can actually observe vs. what you're imagining
- Current conditions vs. theoretical possibilities
- Evidence-based information vs. anxiety-driven assumptions

Practice Tips

- Start with neutral situations to build the skill
- Use it regularly, not just during crisis moments

- Focus on gathering information, not reducing anxiety
- Notice how much evidence contradicts your obsessional concerns
- Remember that reality sensing takes practice to become automatic

What to Expect

- Initial discomfort as you notice the gap between obsessional thinking and reality
- Gradual increase in confidence about your ability to assess situations
- Reduced need for compulsive behaviors as you trust sensory evidence
- Improved decision-making based on what's actually happening

Common Mistakes to Avoid

- Using reality sensing as a new compulsion (keep it brief - under 30 seconds)
- Expecting immediate anxiety relief (focus on information gathering)
- Dismissing what you observe because it contradicts obsessional thinking
- Only using the technique during crisis moments instead of regular practice

Homework Instructions

Module 1-3 Homework: Obsessional Sequence Tracking

Your Assignment: Track at least three obsessional episodes over the next week using the Obsessional Sequence Mapping Worksheet.

Instructions:

1. Keep the worksheet easily accessible (phone, purse, desk)
2. Complete it as soon as possible after an obsessional episode
3. Be specific about each stage - avoid general descriptions
4. Focus on one clear episode rather than trying to analyze multiple concerns

What to Track:

- **Trigger:** What specifically started the episode?
- **Doubt:** What was the first "what if" thought?
- **Consequence:** What did your mind say would happen?
- **Anxiety:** How did your body respond?
- **Compulsion:** What did you do to handle the anxiety?

Tips for Success:

- Start with shorter, simpler episodes if longer ones feel overwhelming
- If you can't remember exact details, make notes immediately when episodes occur
- Don't judge yourself for having obsessional thoughts - you're learning to observe them
- Bring completed worksheets to your next session for discussion

Module 4-6 Homework: Evidence vs. Imagination Sorting

Your Assignment: For each obsessional concern that arises, create two lists: "What I Can Actually Observe" and "What I'm Imagining Might Be True."

Instructions:

1. When an obsessional concern arises, pause before taking action
2. List everything you can observe through your senses
3. List everything you're worried might be true but can't actually observe
4. Notice which list is longer and which feels more compelling

Example: *Concern: Kitchen counter might be contaminated*

What I Can Actually Observe:

- Counter appears clean
- No visible stains or residue
- No unusual odors
- Family has been healthy despite using this counter
- I cleaned it yesterday with standard household cleaner

What I'm Imagining Might Be True:

- Invisible bacteria could be present
- Cleaning might not have been thorough enough
- Family could get sick from contamination I can't see
- I might be missing something dangerous

Modules 7-9 Homework: Reality Sensing Practice

Your Assignment: Practice the 5-4-3-2-1 reality sensing technique daily, both during calm moments and when obsessional thinking arises.

Daily Practice Schedule:

- **Morning:** One reality sensing exercise before starting your day
- **Midday:** One exercise during a regular activity
- **Evening:** One exercise before bedtime
- **As needed:** During obsessional episodes

Instructions:

1. Set reminders on your phone for scheduled practice times
2. Use the Reality Sensing Diary to track your experiences
3. Notice how reality sensing affects your perception of obsessional concerns
4. Practice in different environments and situations

What to Notice:

- How much sensory evidence contradicts your obsessional concerns
- The difference between what you can observe vs. what you're imagining
- Changes in anxiety or urgency after reality sensing
- Increased confidence in your ability to assess situations

Modules 10-12 Homework: Alternative Story Development

Your Assignment: For your main obsessional themes, develop evidence-based alternative stories that account for the same observations without requiring compulsive responses.

Instructions:

1. Choose your most frequent obsessional concern
2. Write out your typical obsessional story about this concern
3. Identify the reasoning errors in your obsessional story
4. Create an alternative story based solely on observable evidence
5. Test the alternative story by using it to guide your behavior

Alternative Story Template:

Obsessional Story: "I'm concerned about _____ because _____. If I don't _____, then _____ might happen, which would mean _____."

Evidence-Based Alternative: "The observable facts are _____. A reasonable response to these facts is _____. Normal people in this situation would _____."

General Homework Guidelines

Time Commitment:

- Plan 15-20 minutes daily for homework activities
- Don't let homework become a new compulsion
- Focus on learning rather than perfect completion

When You Struggle:

- Do what you can rather than avoiding homework entirely
- Bring questions and challenges to your next session

- Remember that struggling with homework is part of the learning process
- Modify assignments if they feel overwhelming

Recording Your Experience:
- Use the provided forms and worksheets
- Note both successes and challenges
- Track patterns and changes over time
- Bring completed homework to each session

Relapse Prevention Planning Guide

Understanding Relapse vs. Setbacks

Normal Setbacks:
- Brief return of obsessional thoughts during stress
- Occasional use of old compulsive behaviors
- Temporary increases in anxiety during life changes
- Questioning whether you're applying techniques correctly

Concerning Relapse Signs:
- Return to pre-treatment levels of obsessional behavior
- Loss of insight into reasoning errors
- Abandoning I-CBT techniques for weeks at a time
- Significant functional impairment returning

Early Warning Sign Recognition

Behavioral Warning Signs:

- Gradual increases in checking, cleaning, or avoidance
- "Just to be safe" thinking returning
- Spending more time on routine activities
- Asking for reassurance more frequently

Cognitive Warning Signs:

- Decreased trust in sensory evidence
- Increased focus on theoretical possibilities
- Return of "what if" thinking patterns
- Difficulty distinguishing evidence from imagination

Emotional Warning Signs:

- Increased anxiety about normal uncertainty
- Feeling overwhelmed by routine decisions
- Return of urgency about minor concerns
- Loss of confidence in your judgment

Your Personal Warning Signs: (Fill in based on your experience)

1. _____
2. _____
3. _____

Emergency Response Plan

When You Notice Warning Signs:

Step 1: Immediate Response

- Use reality sensing to assess the current situation

- Review your inference chain mapping skills
- Apply evidence evaluation techniques
- Resist the urge to perform compulsions

Step 2: Review and Practice

- Review your I-CBT handouts and worksheets
- Practice techniques you found most helpful during treatment
- Use your alternative stories for current concerns
- Return to daily reality sensing practice

Step 3: Seek Support

- Contact your therapist for a booster session
- Reach out to trusted friends or family members
- Consider attending an OCD support group
- Use online I-CBT resources for reinforcement

Step 4: Professional Help If warning signs persist for more than two weeks or worsen significantly:

- Schedule an appointment with your I-CBT therapist
- Consider intensive treatment if available
- Discuss with your doctor if medication changes might be helpful
- Don't wait until symptoms return to pre-treatment levels

Ongoing Maintenance Strategies

Daily Practices:

- Continue using reality sensing regularly

- Maintain awareness of your reasoning patterns
- Practice evidence-based decision-making
- Stay connected to your authentic values and goals

Weekly Practices:
- Review your progress and celebrate successes
- Practice challenging situations using I-CBT techniques
- Connect with supportive people who understand your recovery
- Engage in meaningful activities beyond symptom management

Monthly Practices:
- Complete Y-BOCS and ICQ-EV assessments to track progress
- Review your relapse prevention plan and update as needed
- Reflect on how your life has improved since treatment
- Set new goals for continued growth and development

Stress Management: High stress often triggers obsessional thinking. Maintain:
- Regular sleep schedule
- Healthy eating habits
- Regular exercise or physical activity
- Stress reduction practices (meditation, hobbies, relaxation)
- Social connections and support systems

Remember:

- Recovery is a process, not a destination
- Occasional setbacks are normal and expected
- You have skills and tools to handle challenges
- Professional support is available when needed
- Your life can continue improving beyond symptom management

Emergency Contacts:

Therapist: _____
Crisis Line: _____
Trusted Friend/Family: _____
Support Group: _____

Appendix C: Case Studies and Clinical Examples

Complete Case Study: Contamination OCD (Sarah, 28)

Background Information

Sarah is a 28-year-old marketing professional and mother of two young children (ages 3 and 5). She was referred for I-CBT after three previous attempts at traditional CBT/ERP treatment resulted in minimal improvement and high dropout rates due to the distress of exposure exercises. Her contamination obsessions began during her first pregnancy but worsened significantly after her second child was born.

Presenting Concerns

Sarah's primary symptoms center on contamination fears that interfere significantly with daily functioning:

- Elaborate hand-washing rituals lasting 10-15 minutes, performed 15-20 times daily
- Kitchen cleaning routines requiring 2-3 hours each evening
- Avoidance of public restrooms, playgrounds, and other "contaminated" environments
- Excessive concern about family illness prevention
- Intrusive thoughts about being responsible for making her children sick

Her Y-BOCS score at intake was 26 (severe range), and her ICQ-EV score was 34, indicating significant inferential confusion.

Case Conceptualization

Vulnerable Self-Theme: Sarah's obsessions center on maternal competence and family protection. Her feared possible self is "the negligent mother who fails to protect her children and causes them unnecessary suffering."

Primary Reasoning Errors:

- Inverse inference: Starting with contamination possibilities rather than observable evidence

- Irrelevant association: Applying medical contamination information to normal household situations

- Category error: Using hospital-level hygiene standards for domestic environments

- Sensory distrust: Dismissing clear evidence of cleanliness in favor of imagined contamination

Obsessional Narrative: "Dangerous germs exist everywhere and could harm my children through my carelessness. Normal cleaning standards aren't sufficient to protect them from serious illness. As a responsible mother, I must do everything possible to prevent contamination, even if it seems excessive to others."

Treatment Course

Sessions 1-3: Assessment and Education Sarah quickly grasped the obsessional sequence concept, identifying her pattern: Environmental trigger → contamination possibility → family illness fear → maternal failure anxiety → extensive cleaning. She showed high insight, acknowledging that her behaviors seemed excessive while feeling unable to resist them.

Sessions 4-6: Reasoning Error Recognition Sarah readily identified reasoning errors in hypothetical scenarios but struggled to apply this recognition to her own thinking. She had difficulty accepting that medical contamination information didn't apply to her home environment, arguing that "good mothers don't take chances with their children's health."

Sessions 7-9: Vulnerable Theme Work Exploring her maternal competence themes proved emotionally challenging. Sarah revealed perfectionist expectations inherited from her own mother and intense guilt about any perceived failures in child care. Module 5 work (OCD is 100% imaginary) produced significant breakthrough when she realized her contamination concerns lacked any observable evidence.

Sessions 10-12: Reality Sensing and Evidence Evaluation Sarah mastered reality sensing techniques quickly, finding them particularly helpful in kitchen situations. She began completing household tasks based on evidence rather than anxiety, reducing cleaning time from 3 hours to 45 minutes within three weeks.

Sessions 13-15: Alternative Story Development Sarah developed evidence-based stories about normal household hygiene: "Typical home environments contain normal bacteria that healthy immune systems handle routinely. Standard cleaning provides adequate protection. Good mothers focus on overall child wellbeing, not perfect contamination prevention."

Sessions 16-18: Integration and Relapse Prevention Final sessions focused on maintaining gains and addressing subtle forms of obsessional thinking that emerged as obvious symptoms decreased. Sarah learned to recognize when "reasonable precautions" were becoming excessive again.

Treatment Outcomes

Symptom Improvement:

- Y-BOCS score decreased from 26 to 8 (minimal symptoms)

- ICQ-EV score decreased from 34 to 12 (normal range)
- Hand-washing reduced to normal frequency and duration
- Kitchen cleaning time reduced by 75%
- Return to previously avoided activities with children

Functional Improvements:

- Increased time available for family activities
- Reduced family stress and accommodation
- Return to social activities and public outings
- Improved work performance due to reduced preoccupation
- Enhanced confidence in parenting abilities

Six-Month Follow-Up: Sarah maintained her gains with occasional minor setbacks during high-stress periods. She used booster sessions at 3 and 6 months to reinforce techniques and address new challenges. Her Y-BOCS score remained in the minimal range (6-8).

Key Learning Points:

- Vulnerable theme work was crucial for lasting improvement
- Reality sensing provided immediate practical benefits
- Alternative story development helped integrate new thinking patterns
- Family education enhanced treatment compliance and reduced accommodation

Complete Case Study: Checking Behaviors (Mark, 35)

Background Information

Mark is a 35-year-old software engineer who lives alone in a downtown apartment. His checking behaviors began in college but intensified significantly after a break-in occurred in his apartment building two years ago. Despite the building's improved security, Mark's checking behaviors continued escalating until they consumed 2-3 hours daily.

Presenting Concerns

Mark's obsessions focus on security and safety checking:

- Door lock checking requiring 15-20 repetitions before leaving home
- Stove and appliance checking taking 30-45 minutes each evening
- Window and security system verification multiple times nightly
- Extensive car door and alarm checking
- Intrusive thoughts about being responsible for preventable disasters

His Y-BOCS score was 22 (moderate-severe range), with ICQ-EV score of 28.

Case Conceptualization

Vulnerable Self-Theme: Mark's obsessions center on competence and responsibility. His feared possible self is "the careless, irresponsible person who causes disasters through inadequate attention to safety."

Primary Reasoning Errors:

- Inverse inference: Starting with disaster possibilities rather than current security evidence

- Category error: Applying high-security facility standards to residential situations

- Over-reliance on possibility: Treating theoretical security breaches as probable concerns

- Sensory distrust: Questioning clear evidence that doors are locked and appliances are off

Obsessional Narrative: "Serious accidents and security breaches result from momentary carelessness. Competent, responsible people anticipate and prevent all reasonably possible disasters. The consequences of being wrong about safety are too serious to risk normal confidence levels."

Treatment Course

Sessions 1-4: Foundation Building Mark easily understood the inference chain concept and quickly mapped his checking sequences. He showed good insight but argued that his security concerns were more realistic than typical OCD presentations, given the previous break-in in his building.

Sessions 5-8: Challenging Overvalued Ideation Mark demonstrated moderate overvalued ideation about security threats. Treatment required careful balance between acknowledging realistic security considerations and helping him recognize obsessional overcautiousness. Collaborative evidence evaluation helped him distinguish between reasonable precautions and excessive checking.

Sessions 9-12: Reality Sensing Implementation Mark initially resisted reality sensing, arguing that visual evidence wasn't sufficient for important security decisions. Gradual practice helped him recognize that sensory evidence was more reliable than anxiety-driven doubt. He learned to trust what he could see and feel about door locks and appliance positions.

Sessions 13-16: Behavioral Change As Mark's confidence in reality sensing grew, his checking behaviors decreased dramatically. He reduced door checking from 20 repetitions to 2-3, and appliance checking from 45 minutes to 5 minutes. This rapid improvement surprised him and increased motivation for continued work.

Sessions 17-20: Advanced Integration Later sessions addressed subtle forms of checking that emerged as obvious behaviors decreased. Mark learned to recognize mental checking and "just to be sure" behaviors that maintained his obsessional patterns. Relapse prevention focused on maintaining appropriate security practices without obsessional excess.

Treatment Outcomes

Symptom Improvement:

- Y-BOCS score decreased from 22 to 5 (minimal symptoms)
- ICQ-EV score decreased from 28 to 9 (normal range)
- Checking time reduced by 90%
- Elimination of repetitive checking behaviors
- Return to normal leaving and bedtime routines

Functional Improvements:

- Regained 2-3 hours daily for meaningful activities
- Reduced chronic lateness due to checking delays
- Improved work punctuality and productivity
- Enhanced social life through reliable scheduling
- Increased confidence in independent living skills

Key Learning Points:

- Overvalued ideation required modified approach emphasizing collaboration
- Reality sensing was most effective intervention for this presentation
- Gradual exposure to reduced checking built confidence in technique
- Addressing competence themes prevented symptom substitution

Complete Case Study: "Pure O" Presentation (Lisa, 24)

Background Information

Lisa is a 24-year-old recent college graduate working at a marketing firm. Her OCD presentation primarily involves intrusive thoughts about harming others and sexual content, with minimal observable compulsions. She was referred for I-CBT after six months of traditional CBT showed limited improvement and increased distress from exposure exercises focusing on her intrusive thoughts.

Presenting Concerns

Lisa's symptoms center on unwanted intrusive thoughts:

- Intrusive images of harming coworkers or family members
- Unwanted sexual thoughts about inappropriate people or situations
- Obsessive analysis of her thoughts and their meaning
- Mental checking and reviewing to ensure she doesn't want to act on thoughts
- Avoidance of situations that trigger intrusive thoughts

- Intense guilt and shame about thought content

Her Y-BOCS score was 20 (moderate range), with ICQ-EV score of 31.

Case Conceptualization

Vulnerable Self-Theme: Lisa's obsessions focus on moral character and identity. Her feared possible self is "the dangerous, perverted person who has evil desires and could harm innocent people."

Primary Reasoning Errors:

- Inverse inference: Starting with feared identity possibilities rather than behavioral evidence
- Category error: Applying thought-action fusion beliefs inappropriately
- Irrelevant association: Connecting random thoughts to character assessment
- Over-reliance on possibility: Treating thought occurrence as evidence of desire or intent

Obsessional Narrative: "Having disturbing thoughts means something about my character and desires. Normal people don't have such thoughts, so I must be dangerous or perverted. I need to analyze these thoughts carefully to ensure I don't want to act on them."

Treatment Course

Sessions 1-5: Psychoeducation and Normalization Lisa required extensive education about intrusive thought universality and normal vs. obsessional responses to unwanted mental content. Learning that 90% of people experience intrusive thoughts provided significant relief and hope.

Sessions 6-10: Thought-Identity Separation Core work focused on helping Lisa distinguish between having thoughts and endorsing them. Module 5 work was particularly powerful, demonstrating that her concerns about her character lacked any behavioral evidence. She learned that thoughts are mental events, not identity indicators.

Sessions 11-15: Mental Compulsion Recognition Lisa initially denied having compulsions but gradually recognized extensive mental checking, reviewing, and analysis behaviors. She learned to identify and interrupt mental rituals just as others interrupt behavioral compulsions.

Sessions 16-20: Values-Based Living Final sessions emphasized living according to actual values rather than trying to control thought content. Lisa engaged in value-congruent activities that provided evidence of her actual character, contradicting her obsessional fears.

Treatment Outcomes

Symptom Improvement:

- Y-BOCS score decreased from 20 to 7 (minimal symptoms)
- ICQ-EV score decreased from 31 to 11 (normal range)
- Dramatic reduction in mental checking and analysis
- Decreased distress about intrusive thought content
- Return to normal daily activities without avoidance

Functional Improvements:

- Reduced preoccupation allowing focus on work and relationships
- Elimination of thought-triggered avoidance behaviors
- Improved self-confidence and self-compassion

- Enhanced ability to engage in meaningful activities
- Reduced shame and increased willingness to seek support when needed

Key Learning Points:

- "Pure O" presentations respond well to I-CBT reasoning analysis
- Thought-identity separation was crucial intervention
- Mental compulsion recognition required careful assessment
- Values-based living provided positive alternative to thought control

---

Brief Vignettes for Various Presentations

Religious Scrupulosity - Father Miguel, 45

Miguel, a devoted Catholic and father of three, developed obsessive concerns about blasphemous thoughts and moral perfection. His obsessions included intrusive thoughts during prayer, excessive confession behaviors, and elaborate mental rituals to "cancel out" perceived sins.

I-CBT Application: Treatment focused on distinguishing authentic spiritual practice from obsessional behavior. Miguel learned that intrusive thoughts during prayer were normal mental events, not spiritual failures. Reality sensing helped him recognize when religious practices were driven by anxiety rather than genuine devotion. Collaboration with his priest supported treatment by confirming that obsessive confession was not spiritually beneficial.

Outcome: Miguel returned to normal religious practice within 12 sessions, maintaining his faith while eliminating obsessional behaviors.

Relationship OCD - Jennifer, 29

Jennifer obsessed about her feelings for her boyfriend, constantly analyzing whether she truly loved him and seeking reassurance about their relationship. She spent hours mentally reviewing their interactions and comparing her feelings to idealized romantic love.

I-CBT Application: Treatment revealed that Jennifer was treating emotional uncertainty as dangerous rather than normal. She learned that relationships involve ongoing choice rather than constant feeling verification. Reality sensing focused on behavioral evidence of care and commitment rather than emotional analysis.

Outcome: Jennifer's relationship anxiety decreased significantly as she learned to act based on values rather than feeling certainty.

Health Anxiety - Robert, 52

Robert interpreted normal bodily sensations as signs of serious illness, despite repeated medical reassurance. He spent hours researching symptoms online and seeking medical consultations for minor concerns.

I-CBT Application: Treatment helped Robert distinguish between medical awareness and obsessional hypervigilance. He learned to evaluate health concerns using appropriate evidence rather than worst-case possibility thinking. Reality sensing helped him recognize normal vs. concerning bodily sensations.

Outcome: Robert's medical visits decreased from weekly to appropriate frequency, with improved trust in medical professionals and his own body awareness.

Cultural Diversity in Case Examples

Korean-American Family Dynamics - Grace, 31

Grace's contamination obsessions were complicated by cultural expectations about cleanliness and family responsibility. Her traditional Korean mother supported excessive cleaning behaviors, viewing them as proper feminine conduct rather than symptoms.

Cultural Adaptations:

- Family education sessions explaining OCD vs. cultural cleanliness values
- Respectful exploration of how cultural practices could be maintained without obsessional excess
- Collaboration with culturally knowledgeable supervisor
- Integration of family harmony values with individual recovery

Outcome: Grace reduced obsessional behaviors while maintaining cultural cleanliness practices, with family support for her recovery.

Mexican-American Religious Integration - Carlos, 38

Carlos experienced religious scrupulosity complicated by folk religious practices and extended family involvement in spiritual matters. His obsessions included fears about spiritual contamination and elaborate purification rituals.

Cultural Adaptations:

- Collaboration with culturally informed religious leader
- Distinction between traditional spiritual practices and obsessional behaviors
- Family sessions to address collective responsibility vs. individual symptoms
- Integration of community healing approaches with individual therapy

Outcome: Carlos maintained meaningful spiritual practices while eliminating obsessional rituals, with community support for his recovery.

First-Generation Immigrant Challenges - Amin, 26

Amin, recently immigrated from Somalia, developed checking behaviors around home security due to trauma history and cultural adjustment stress. Language barriers and cultural concepts of mental health complicated treatment.

Cultural Adaptations:

- Use of interpreter services for complex concepts
- Cultural consultant to understand refugee experience and trauma impact
- Modified explanations of reasoning concepts using culturally relevant examples
- Integration with refugee support services for holistic care

Outcome: Amin's security checking decreased significantly with improved cultural adjustment and trauma processing.

These case examples illustrate the flexibility and effectiveness of I-CBT across diverse presentations and populations. The key to successful treatment lies in maintaining core I-CBT principles while adapting presentation and application to individual cultural, religious, and personal factors.

Appendix D: Training Resources and References

Essential Reading List

Core I-CBT Texts

1. O'Connor, K., Aardema, F., & Pélissier, M. C. (2005). *Beyond reasonable doubt: Reasoning processes in obsessive-compulsive disorder and related disorders.* John Wiley & Sons.

2. Aardema, F., & O'Connor, K. (2012). *Handbook of obsessive-compulsive and related disorders.* Academic Press.

3. O'Connor, K. (2020). *Cognitive-behavioral therapy for obsessive-compulsive disorder: An inference-based approach.* Guilford Press.

Foundational Research Articles

4. O'Connor, K., & Robillard, S. (1995). Inference processes in obsessive-compulsive disorder: Some neuropsychological and clinical observations. *Behaviour Research and Therapy, 33*(8), 887-896.

5. Aardema, F., & O'Connor, K. (2003). Seeing white bears that are not there: Inference processes in obsessions. *Journal of Cognitive Psychotherapy, 17*(1), 23-37.

6. O'Connor, K., Aardema, F., Bouthillier, D., Fournier, S., Guay, S., Robillard, S., ... & Tremblay, M. (2005). Evaluation of an inference-based approach to treating

obsessive-compulsive disorder. *Cognitive Behaviour Therapy, 34*(3), 148-163.

Assessment and Measurement

7. Aardema, F., Wu, K. D., Careau, Y., O'Connor, K., Julien, D., & Dennie, S. (2010). The expanded version of the Inferential Confusion Questionnaire: Further development and validation in clinical and non-clinical samples. *Journal of Psychopathology and Behavioral Assessment, 32*(3), 448-462.

8. Pélissier, M. C., O'Connor, K. P., & Dupuis, G. (2009). When doubting becomes excessive: A psychometric analysis of the Inferential Confusion Questionnaire. *Cognitive Therapy and Research, 33*(5), 492-501.

Clinical Applications and Outcomes

9. O'Connor, K., Julien, D., Aardema, F., Robillard, S., Pépin, A. L., Borgeat, F., & Leblanc, V. (2007). Cognitive behaviour therapy and medication in the treatment of obsessive-compulsive disorder: A controlled study. *Canadian Journal of Psychiatry, 52*(7), 424-431.

10. Aardema, F., Kleijer, T., Lavoie, M. E., Menon, M., O'Connor, K., & Doucet, P. (2006). Evaluating the effectiveness of an inference-based approach to obsessive-compulsive disorder: A controlled study. *Clinical Psychology and Psychotherapy, 13*(5), 378-387.

Training Program Directory

University-Based Programs

Université de Montréal - Centre de recherche Fernand-Seguin

- Original I-CBT research and training center

- Offers intensive training workshops and research opportunities
- Contact: Research Center Fernand-Seguin, Montreal, Quebec

Concordia University - Department of Psychology

- Graduate courses in I-CBT theory and application
- Research opportunities with I-CBT faculty
- Contact: Department of Psychology, Montreal, Quebec

Private Training Institutes

International Association for Cognitive Behavioral Therapy (ICBT)

- Annual I-CBT training institutes and workshops
- Certification programs for qualified mental health professionals
- Online and in-person training options

OCD Training School

- Specialized I-CBT training programs
- Modular online training with supervision components
- Cultural adaptation training available

Beck Institute for Cognitive Behavior Therapy

- Integrated CBT training including I-CBT modules
- Advanced practitioner workshops
- Supervision and consultation services

Professional Development Organizations

Association for Behavioral and Cognitive Therapies (ABCT)

- Annual conference I-CBT presentations and workshops
- Special interest group for OCD and related disorders
- Continuing education credits available

International OCD Foundation (IOCDF)

- Annual conference with I-CBT training tracks
- Regional workshops and training opportunities
- Therapist referral directory for I-CBT practitioners

Professional Organizations

Primary Organizations

International Association for Cognitive Behavioral Therapy (AICBT)

- Global organization promoting I-CBT research and practice
- Training standards and certification programs
- Annual conferences and research publications

International OCD Foundation (IOCDF)

- Leading organization for OCD research, treatment, and advocacy
- Professional member directory and referral services
- Training and educational resources for clinicians

Association for Behavioral and Cognitive Therapies (ABCT)

- Professional organization for cognitive-behavioral practitioners

- Special interest groups for OCD and anxiety disorders
- Research journals and continuing education opportunities

Regional Organizations

Canadian Association for Cognitive and Behavioural Therapies (CACBT)

- Canadian organization promoting CBT and I-CBT practice
- Provincial chapters with local training opportunities
- Bilingual resources and cultural adaptation support

European Association for Behavioural and Cognitive Therapies (EABCT)

- European network of CBT practitioners and researchers
- I-CBT special interest groups and training initiatives
- Multilingual resources and cultural applications

Online Resources and Communities

Educational Websites

ICBT.online

- Comprehensive I-CBT training platform
- Self-paced modules with video demonstrations
- Progress tracking and competency assessment tools

International OCD Foundation (iocdf.org)

- Extensive educational resources about OCD and treatments
- Treatment provider directory including I-CBT specialists
- Support group listings and peer support resources

Association for Behavioral and Cognitive Therapies (abct.org)
- Professional resources and training opportunities
- Research databases and clinical practice guidelines
- Special interest group information and networking

Professional Discussion Forums

ABCT Community Platform
- Professional discussion forums for CBT practitioners
- I-CBT special interest group discussions
- Case consultation and peer support opportunities

International CBT Network
- Global network of cognitive-behavioral practitioners
- Cultural adaptation discussions and resources
- Research collaboration opportunities

Social Media and Networking

LinkedIn Professional Groups
- Cognitive Behavioral Therapy Professionals
- OCD Treatment and Research Network
- I-CBT Practitioners and Researchers

Training and Supervision Platforms

TheraNest Professional Development
- Online supervision and consultation services
- Video platform for session review and feedback

- Professional development tracking tools

PsychWire Training Network

- Continuing education courses in I-CBT
- Live webinars and recorded training sessions
- Professional networking and mentorship opportunities

Comprehensive Glossary of I-CBT Terms

Cognitive Fusion The blending of primary and secondary inferences until they feel equally real and urgent, making it difficult to distinguish between different levels of reasoning.

Cross-over Point The specific moment in obsessional thinking when reasoning shifts from evidence-based to imagination-based, marking the transition from normal to obsessional thinking.

Feared Possible Self The dreaded identity that a person desperately wants to avoid becoming, which motivates obsessional behaviors as attempts to prevent this outcome.

ICQ-EV (Inferential Confusion Questionnaire-Expanded Version) A validated assessment tool measuring the degree to which individuals rely on imagination rather than evidence when making decisions.

Inference Chain The sequential progression from trigger through doubt, consequences, anxiety, and compulsion that characterizes obsessional episodes.

Inferential Confusion The core mechanism of OCD involving reliance on imagination and theoretical possibilities rather than observable evidence for decision-making.

Inverse Inference A reasoning error where thinking starts with feared outcomes and works backward to current concerns, rather than starting with evidence and reasoning forward.

OCD Bubble The alternate psychological reality created by obsessional thinking, where possibilities feel more compelling than probabilities and imagination overrides evidence.

Obsessional Doubt A specific type of uncertainty that persists despite contradictory evidence and regenerates itself rather than being resolved through investigation.

Obsessional Narrative The complete story that explains why obsessional concerns are important and compulsive responses are necessary, typically containing multiple reasoning errors.

Primary Inference The initial doubt or "what if" thought that represents the cross-over from reality-based to imagination-based thinking.

Reality Sensing Techniques for staying connected to observable evidence rather than getting pulled into imagination-based concerns, typically using systematic sensory awareness.

Reasoning Device Specific cognitive errors that OCD uses to make imagination-based concerns feel realistic and urgent, including inverse inference, category errors, and sensory distrust.

Secondary Inference Subsequent thoughts that build on primary inferences, typically involving increasingly catastrophic consequences and identity themes.

Sensory Distrust A reasoning error involving dismissal of clear sensory evidence in favor of imagined possibilities or theoretical concerns.

Vulnerable Self-Theme Core identity areas where individuals are particularly sensitive to doubt because they connect to fundamental values, relationships, and sense of adequacy.

This comprehensive training resource appendix provides the foundation for developing expertise in I-CBT practice. The combination of established research, practical tools, ongoing education opportunities, and professional networking creates a robust support system for practitioners committed to mastering this effective approach to treating obsessive-compulsive disorder.

Final Integration Points

This complete training manual represents the current state of knowledge in I-CBT theory and practice. As the field continues to develop, practitioners should remain committed to ongoing learning, ethical practice, and contribution to the evidence base through clinical work and research participation.

The journey from novice to expert practitioner requires patience, persistence, and commitment to the reasoning-based principles that make I-CBT uniquely effective. By maintaining focus on evidence rather than anxiety, possibility rather than probability, and authentic values rather than obsessional concerns, practitioners can help clients achieve lasting freedom from the reasoning errors that create obsessional suffering.

Success in I-CBT practice ultimately depends on the same principles we teach clients: trusting evidence over imagination, making decisions based on observable reality rather than theoretical possibilities, and maintaining confidence in our ability to navigate uncertainty using the best information available. These principles serve both practitioner and client in the shared journey toward reasoning-based living.

Reference

- Aardema, F., Emmelkamp, P. M. G., & O'Connor, K. (2005). Inferential confusion, cognitive change and treatment outcome in obsessive–compulsive disorder. *Clinical Psychology & Psychotherapy, 12*(5), 337–345. https://doi.org/10.1002/cpp.464

- Aardema, F., & O'Connor, K. (2007). The menace within: Obsessions and the self. *Journal of Cognitive Psychotherapy, 21*(3), 182–197. https://doi.org/10.1891/088983907781494573

- Aardema, F., & O'Connor, K. (2016). The inference-based approach to obsessive–compulsive disorder: A comprehensive review of its etiological model, treatment efficacy, and model of change. *Journal of Affective Disorders, 202*, 187–196.

- Aardema, F., O'Connor, K., Côté, S., & Taillon, A. (2010). Virtual reality induces dissociation and lowers sense of presence in objective reality. *Cyberpsychology, Behavior, and Social Networking, 13*(4), 429–435. https://doi.org/10.1089/cyber.2009.0164

- Aardema, F., O'Connor, K., Emmelkamp, P. M. G., Marchand, A., & Todorov, C. (2005). Inferential confusion in obsessive–compulsive disorder: The Inferential Confusion Questionnaire. *Behaviour Research and Therapy, 43*(3), 293–308.

- Aardema, F., Wu, K. D., Careau, Y., O'Connor, K., Julien, D., & Dennie, S. (2010). The expanded version of the

Inferential Confusion Questionnaire: Further development and validation in clinical and non-clinical samples. *Journal of Psychopathology and Behavioral Assessment, 32*(3), 448–462.

- Clark, D. A. (2004). *Cognitive-Behavioral Therapy for OCD*. Guilford Press.

- Clark, D. A., & O'Connor, K. (2005). Thinking is believing: Ego-dystonic intrusive thoughts in obsessive–compulsive disorder. In D. A. Clark (Ed.), *Intrusive thoughts in clinical disorders* (pp. 145–174). Guilford Press.

- Eisen, J. L., Phillips, K. A., Baer, L., Beer, D. A., Atala, K. D., & Rasmussen, S. A. (1998). The Brown Assessment of Beliefs Scale: Reliability and validity. *American Journal of Psychiatry, 155*(1), 102–108.

- Kozak, M. J., & Foa, E. B. (1994). Obsessions, overvalued ideas, and delusions in obsessive–compulsive disorder. *Behaviour Research and Therapy, 32*(3), 343–353.

- O'Connor, K. (2002). Intrusions and inferences in obsessive–compulsive disorder. *Clinical Psychology & Psychotherapy, 9*(1), 38–46. https://doi.org/10.1002/cpp.303

- O'Connor, K. P., Aardema, F., & Pélissier, M.-C. (2005). *Beyond reasonable doubt: Reasoning processes in obsessive–compulsive disorder and related disorders*. John Wiley & Sons.

- O'Connor, K., Aardema, F., Bouthillier, D., Fournier, S., Guay, S., Robillard, S., ... Tremblay, M. (2005). Evaluation of an inference-based approach to treating obsessive–compulsive disorder. *Cognitive Behaviour Therapy, 34*(3), 148–163.

- O'Connor, K., Aardema, F., Robillard, S., Guay, S., Pélissier, M.-C., Todorov, C., ... Pitre, D. (2006). Cognitive behaviour therapy and medication in the treatment of obsessive–compulsive disorder. *Acta Psychiatrica Scandinavica, 113*(5), 408–419. https://doi.org/10.1111/j.1600-0447.2006.00767.x

- O'Connor, K., Koszegi, N., Aardema, F., van Niekerk, J., & Taillon, A. (2009). An inference-based approach to treating obsessive–compulsive disorders. *Cognitive and Behavioral Practice, 16*(4), 420–429. https://doi.org/10.1016/j.cbpra.2009.04.002

- Pélissier, M.-C., & O'Connor, K. P. (2002). Deductive and inductive reasoning in obsessive–compulsive disorder. *British Journal of Clinical Psychology, 41*(1), 15–27. https://doi.org/10.1348/014466502163769

- Pinto, A., Mancebo, M. C., Eisen, J. L., Pagano, M. E., & Rasmussen, S. A. (2006). The Brown Longitudinal Obsessive Compulsive Study: Clinical features at intake. *Journal of Clinical Psychiatry, 67*(5), 703–711.

- Rachman, S. (1997). A cognitive theory of obsessions. *Behaviour Research and Therapy, 35*(9), 793–802.

- Rachman, S., & de Silva, P. (1978). Abnormal and normal obsessions. *Behaviour Research and Therapy, 16*(4), 233–248.

- Rassin, E., & Koster, E. (2003). The correlation between thought–action fusion and religiosity in a normal sample. *Behaviour Research and Therapy, 41*(3), 361–368.

- Salkovskis, P. M. (1985). Obsessional–compulsive problems: A cognitive–behavioural analysis. *Behaviour Research and Therapy, 23*(5), 571–583.

- Salkovskis, P. M. (1999). Understanding and treating obsessive–compulsive disorder. *Behaviour Research and Therapy, 37*(Suppl 1), S29–S52.

- Taillon, A., O'Connor, K., Dupuis, G., & Lavoie, M. (2013). Inference-based therapy for body dysmorphic disorder. *Clinical Psychology & Psychotherapy, 20*(1), 67–76. https://doi.org/10.1002/cpp.767

- Tallis, F., Eysenck, M., & Mathews, A. (1991). Elevated evidence requirements and worry. *Personality and Individual Differences, 12*(1), 21–27.

- Veale, D. (2002). Over-valued ideas: A conceptual analysis. *Behaviour Research and Therapy, 40*(4), 383–400.

- Visser, H. A., van Oppen, P., van Megen, H. J., Eikelenboom, M., & van Balkom, A. J. L. M. (2014). Obsessive–compulsive disorder; chronic versus non-chronic symptoms. *Journal of Affective Disorders, 152*, 169–174. https://doi.org/10.1016/j.jad.2013.09.004

- Whittal, M. L., Thordarson, D. S., & McLean, P. D. (2005). Treatment of obsessive–compulsive disorder: Cognitive behavior therapy vs. exposure and response prevention. *Behaviour Research and Therapy, 43*(12), 1559–1576.

- Woody, S. R., Whittal, M. L., & McLean, P. D. (2011). Mechanisms of symptom reduction in treatment for obsessions. *Journal of Consulting and Clinical Psychology, 79*(5), 653–664.

- Wu, K. D., Aardema, F., & O'Connor, K. P. (2009). Inferential confusion, obsessive beliefs, and obsessive–compulsive symptoms: A replication and extension. *Journal of Anxiety Disorders, 23*(6), 746–752. https://doi.org/10.1016/j.janxdis.2009.02.017

- Öst, L. G., Havnen, A., Hansen, B., & Kvale, G. (2015). Cognitive behavioral treatments of obsessive–compulsive disorder: A systematic review and meta-analysis of studies published 1993–2014. *Clinical Psychology Review, 40*, 156–169.

www.ingramcontent.com/pod-product-compliance
Lightning Source LLC
LaVergne TN
LVHW050250170426
836586LV00034B/383